Intermittent Fasting

Metabolic Timing, Body Composition, and Sustainable Health

NATHAN REED

Published by Perennial Publishing

Paperback ISBN: 978-1-971996-09-7
Hardcover ISBN: 978-1-971996-10-3
E-book ISBN: 978-1-971996-11-0

This book is intended for educational and informational purposes only. It does not constitute medical, nutritional, or health advice. The author and publisher make no representations or warranties regarding the completeness or accuracy of the information contained herein. Readers are responsible for their own health decisions and are encouraged to consult qualified healthcare professionals before making changes to diet, fasting practices, supplementation, exercise, or lifestyle. The author and publisher shall not be held liable for any loss, injury, or damages arising from the use of this material.

Contents

Introduction

Intermittent fasting is a feeding timing structure.

It refers to the deliberate organization of eating and non-eating intervals within a repeating temporal frame. Most commonly, this frame aligns with a twenty-four-hour circadian cycle, though it may also extend across multiple days. The defining characteristic is not the duration of abstention or the number of meals consumed, but the patterned distribution of energy intake across time.

Intermittent fasting is therefore structural rather than prescriptive. It describes how feeding is arranged—not what is eaten, how much is eaten, or why it is eaten. It does not require adherence to a named protocol. It does not imply a specific macronutrient composition. It does not prescribe caloric intake. It defines only the temporal boundary between feeding and non-feeding states.

Popular discourse often equates intermittent fasting with specific formats—sixteen hours of fasting followed by eight hours of eating, one meal per day, alternate-day fasting, or other branded configurations. These formats are instantiations of timing structure: examples, not the definition. The concept remains intact regardless of the specific ratio applied.

This distinction matters because fixation on format obscures the underlying variable. When attention centers on whether a window is six hours or eight, the conversation shifts from structural principle to procedural allegiance. The core variable is timing distribution. The numerical configuration is secondary.

It is also essential to separate intermittent fasting from caloric restriction.

Caloric restriction refers to sustained reduction in total energy intake relative to energy expenditure. It is quantitative. Intermittent fasting is temporal. An individual may compress intake into a shortened window while maintaining total daily calories. Conversely, one may eat throughout the day while reducing total calories.

Timing and quantity operate as independent variables. They frequently interact, but they are not interchangeable. Confusion arises when outcomes attributable to reduced intake are credited to timing alone, or when timing is assumed to override energy balance.

Body mass and body composition are governed by cumulative energy balance over time. Intermittent fasting can influence that balance indirectly by shaping appetite patterns, meal frequency, and behavioral containment. It does not remove the requirement that intake and expenditure determine net energy storage or mobilization.

When feeding occurs, the organism enters a fed state characterized by nutrient influx and hormonal response. Insulin rises in proportion to carbohydrate and, to a lesser degree, protein intake. Glucose is directed toward immediate oxidation or glycogen storage. Lipolysis is suppressed when circulating energy is abundant. This state persists for several hours following a meal, depending on its size and composition.

When feeding ceases and circulating nutrients decline, insulin levels fall. The organism transitions toward a post-absorptive state. Glycogen stores are gradually utilized. Lipolysis increases. Fatty acids contribute more substantially to energy production. If fasting extends further, ketone production may increase as an alternative substrate pathway.

These shifts occur daily, regardless of whether one practices intermittent fasting. The human organism continuously oscillates between fed and post-absorptive metabolism. Intermittent fasting modifies the duration and sequencing of these oscillations.

A compressed feeding window lengthens the uninterrupted post-absorptive interval. A dispersed eating pattern shortens it. Neither pattern eliminates the fundamental rhythm; both reorganize its proportions.

Understanding intermittent fasting as a timing structure clarifies its scope. It does not introduce a metabolic state unknown to human physiology. It redistributes temporal exposure to existing states. The physiological processes involved—insulin secretion, glycogen turnover, lipolysis, substrate switching—are not unique to fasting protocols. They are features of normal metabolism arranged differently across time.

This arrangement has implications. Duration of insulin exposure influences how long the organism remains in a predominantly storage-oriented condition. Duration of post-absorptive intervals influences the extent to which endogenous substrates are mobilized between meals. However, these implications are modulated by total intake, activity level, sleep integrity, and prior adaptation.

Intermittent fasting is therefore best understood as a modulation of metabolic rhythm rather than a categorical shift in metabolic identity.
It does not activate a hidden pathway unavailable under other feeding distributions. It alters temporal emphasis.

Because the definition centers on timing, intermittent fasting cannot be evaluated solely by its external format. Two individuals may follow the same nominal schedule yet experience different metabolic realities based on meal composition, caloric load, stress exposure, and sleep quality. Conversely, two individuals with different window lengths may produce similar physiological outcomes if total intake and recovery conditions are comparable.

No moral dimension is embedded in the structure itself. Eating earlier or later in the day does not confer virtue or deficiency. Extending or shortening a fasting interval does not signal discipline or failure. The body responds to inputs according to biological parameters, not ideological ones.

This variable modifies exposure time to feeding and fasting states. It does not determine the total energy entering the system. It does not inherently specify food quality. It does not guarantee metabolic improvement. It does not inherently degrade function.

It organizes time.

From this foundation, subsequent sections will examine how that organization interacts with broader physiological and behavioral systems.

Intermittent fasting does not carry intrinsic directionality. Its effects are conditional.

Any feeding structure interacts with a living system already shaped by prior stress exposure, sleep patterns, training demands, endocrine environment, and energy availability. The same timing arrangement can stabilize one organism and strain another. The structure itself is neutral; the outcome emerges from context.

Metabolic flexibility is one central determinant of that context. Metabolic flexibility refers to the organism's ability to shift between fuel sources—primarily glucose and fatty acids—without excessive physiological disruption. A flexible system transitions between feeding and non-feeding states with minimal volatility in energy, mood, or performance. A less flexible system may exhibit exaggerated hunger signals, cognitive decline, irritability, or stress-hormone elevation when fasting intervals lengthen.

When metabolic flexibility is robust, compressed feeding windows may be tolerated without significant destabilization. When flexibility is constrained—due to chronic overfeeding, prolonged dieting, sleep restriction, or high stress load—the same compression may amplify compensatory responses. These responses are not signs of moral weakness; they are signals of adaptive strain.

Stress load further modulates response. Physiological stress arises not only from external events but from cumulative demands placed on recovery systems. Psychological pressure, high training volumes, caloric deficit, and sleep disruption all contribute. Intermittent fasting introduced into a system already carrying elevated stress may increase allostatic burden. Cortisol exposure may extend. Resting heart-rate variability may decline. Subjective fatigue may intensify.

In contrast, when overall stress load is moderate and recovery systems are intact, similar timing patterns may be integrated without measurable disruption. The distinction lies not in the structure alone, but in the total burden borne by the organism.

Sleep integrity is another critical variable. Sleep regulates glucose tolerance, appetite hormones, and autonomic balance. Shortened or fragmented sleep alters ghrelin and leptin signaling, increases perceived hunger, and impairs insulin sensitivity. In this context, fasting intervals may feel more difficult, and feeding compression may provoke larger swings in appetite. Reduced sleep also diminishes recovery capacity, narrowing the adaptive range within which timing adjustments can be absorbed.

When sleep is stable and circadian rhythms are aligned, metabolic oscillations are more predictable. Timing structures may harmonize with these rhythms or conflict with them depending on scheduling demands. Late-night feeding compression in the presence of circadian misalignment produces different physiological signals than similar compression aligned with daylight hours. The structure remains the same; the interaction shifts.

Underlying all of these variables is the background law of energy balance. Over extended time frames, body mass and tissue distribution reflect the relationship between energy intake and expenditure. Timing influences distribution and perception, not total balance. A compressed window that leads to a consistent energy deficit may reduce mass. The same window accompanied by energy compensation may not.

Adaptive ranges define how far a system can shift without destabilization. Within these ranges, variability is tolerated. Beyond them, threshold responses emerge. These responses may include persistent fatigue, disrupted menstrual cycles, suppressed libido, impaired training recovery, or increased preoccupation with food. Such patterns indicate that the timing structure, in combination with other variables, has exceeded the organism's current capacity.

One instability pattern frequently observed is compensatory overeating within the feeding window. Prolonged fasting may heighten hunger intensity to a degree that intake becomes concentrated and accelerated once eating begins. Total energy may equal or exceed prior levels, accompanied by increased gastrointestinal discomfort or glycemic volatility. The fasting interval did not inherently cause instability; it interacted with appetite regulation and stress load to produce it.

A second instability pattern involves chronic low energy availability masked by adherence to a timing structure. When feeding compression coincides with high activity demands and insufficient total intake, physiological systems may downregulate. Resting energy expenditure can decline. Thyroid signaling may shift. Reproductive hormones may suppress. These changes represent adaptive conservation rather than malfunction, yet they are often misinterpreted as metabolic "damage." The timing pattern becomes the visible variable, while total energy sufficiency remains the underlying driver.

Universal claims frequently obscure this contextual variability. Assertions that intermittent fasting "works for everyone" overlook differences in metabolic flexibility, sleep quality, and workload. Equally categorical claims that fasting "damages metabolism" ignore the adaptive resilience of organisms operating within adequate energy and recovery conditions. Both positions project singular outcomes onto heterogeneous systems.

Capacity-related constraints shape response in quieter ways as well. Adolescents undergoing growth, individuals with high-volume endurance training, pregnant or postpartum women, and those recovering from prolonged dieting often operate with narrower margins for energy restriction. In these contexts, extended fasting intervals may more readily encroach upon recovery requirements. The same structure applied to a sedentary adult with stable intake and sleep may carry different implications. Capacity is not static; it shifts across life stages and stress exposures.

Identical timing structures can therefore produce divergent outcomes because no two systems begin from identical baselines. Basal metabolic rate differs. Hormonal milieu differs. Sleep debt differs. Psychological relationships to food differ. Social environments differ. The structure interacts with all of these variables simultaneously.

It can consolidate intake and reduce grazing behavior in one environment. It can amplify rigidity and physiological strain in another. It can coexist with adequate recovery or compound existing deficits.

The question is not whether intermittent fasting is inherently good or bad. The relevant inquiry concerns the state of the system receiving it and the cumulative load under which it operates.

Intermittent fasting functions within adaptive thresholds shaped by flexibility, stress, sleep, and energy sufficiency, and its outcomes reflect the conditions under which it is imposed.

Human metabolism operates within circadian architecture that organizes hormonal secretion, substrate tolerance, and digestive readiness across the day.

Circadian biology coordinates metabolic readiness. Insulin sensitivity is generally higher earlier in the biological day and declines toward evening. Cortisol follows a diurnal rise after waking and tapers as the day progresses. Melatonin secretion signals transition toward nocturnal physiology, influencing glucose handling and digestive efficiency. These cycles create windows of relative metabolic advantage and disadvantage that repeat with regularity.

Feeding events intersect with these rhythms.

When meals occur, insulin rises to facilitate nutrient storage and distribution. The duration and frequency of these elevations depend on how often and how densely energy is consumed. A pattern of frequent meals distributes insulin exposure more evenly across waking hours. A compressed feeding window concentrates insulin elevations into a shorter span, leaving longer uninterrupted intervals at lower baseline levels.

The distinction is not about whether insulin rises—it does whenever food is consumed—but about how long the organism remains in an elevated state across a full cycle. Timing alters cumulative exposure across time without altering the fundamental role insulin plays.

Glycogen turnover reflects similar temporal organization. Liver glycogen stores fluctuate according to feeding and fasting intervals. After carbohydrate ingestion, glycogen is replenished. During post-absorptive periods, it is gradually depleted to maintain blood glucose stability. If feeding intervals are shorter and more frequent, glycogen stores are replenished before significant depletion occurs. If feeding intervals are longer, depletion progresses further before restoration.

These oscillations influence substrate availability. When glycogen stores are sufficient and insulin is elevated, glucose predominates as a primary fuel. As insulin declines and glycogen decreases, lipolysis increases, and fatty acids contribute more significantly to energy production. If fasting extends beyond glycogen depletion thresholds, ketone production may rise incrementally.

Metabolic switching—the transition between predominant glucose utilization and increased reliance on fatty acids—unfolds along this continuum. It is not a binary event in which the body flips from one exclusive mode to another. Substrates are always mixed; proportions shift gradually in response to hormonal and energetic signals. The duration of post-absorptive intervals influences how far along this continuum the organism travels before feeding resumes.

Feeding frequency shapes hormonal oscillation beyond insulin. Ghrelin, often described as a hunger hormone, rises in anticipation of habitual mealtimes. Its secretion patterns entrain to repeated feeding schedules. If meals occur daily at noon and evening, ghrelin peaks begin to precede those times. When timing shifts, ghrelin rhythms may temporarily misalign until new patterns stabilize.

This entrainment illustrates how timing structures influence subjective experience. Hunger does not arise solely from energy deficit; it also reflects learned temporal expectation. When feeding windows compress, hunger signals may intensify within the narrowed period and diminish outside it as adaptation occurs. Anticipatory appetite can become concentrated rather than evenly distributed.

An example clarifies how altered timing changes hormonal sequencing. Consider an individual who consumes three evenly spaced meals across a twelve-hour waking period. Insulin elevations occur after each meal, separated by moderate intervals. Ghrelin peaks precede each meal, then decline post-consumption. Cortisol follows its diurnal curve largely independent of feeding.

If the same total intake shifts into a six-hour window beginning in late afternoon, hormonal sequencing reorganizes. Insulin elevations become more clustered. The morning hours extend with relatively lower insulin exposure. Ghrelin peaks may intensify in the hours preceding the first meal, then compress around the feeding window. The organism experiences a prolonged post-absorptive interval followed by a condensed fed state. The hormones themselves do not change in function; their timing relative to one another shifts.

Rhythmic alignment or conflict depends on how feeding windows intersect with circadian cues. Early feeding aligned with daylight hours often parallels higher insulin sensitivity and digestive readiness. Late-night feeding, particularly when paired with delayed sleep, can conflict with melatonin-mediated reductions in glucose tolerance. In such cases, identical caloric intake distributed later in the biological evening may result in higher postprandial glucose excursions compared to earlier consumption.

A constraint emerges when feeding compression consistently overlaps with sleep disruption. If the final meal occurs shortly before bedtime, digestive processes and elevated insulin exposure may intersect with the onset of nocturnal hormonal patterns. Sleep fragmentation may increase. Morning appetite cues may shift unpredictably. The instability arises not from compression alone, but from misalignment between feeding rhythm and circadian signaling.

Substrate selection across the day reflects these rhythmic influences. Morning fasted periods may involve greater fatty acid contribution to energy production, particularly after overnight glycogen utilization. Afternoon feeding replenishes stores and shifts substrate mix toward carbohydrate oxidation. The magnitude of these shifts depends on meal composition, activity level, and prior intake, but the pattern remains temporally organized.

Feeding compression reorganizes oscillations by expanding one segment of the cycle and contracting another. The post-absorptive phase lengthens. The fed phase becomes denser. Hormonal peaks cluster. Appetite rhythms entrain to narrower windows. Glycogen depletion may proceed further before replenishment.

None of these processes violate metabolic laws. Energy cannot be generated without substrate. Tissue change still reflects integrated balance over time. What changes is exposure duration—the length of time spent in particular hormonal and substrate states.

Metabolic switching remains a gradient rather than an on–off mechanism. Glycogen turnover continues regardless of feeding window design. Insulin secretion remains proportional to intake. Ghrelin continues to anticipate expected meals. Circadian rhythms persist whether aligned with feeding or not.

Timing matters because it reorganizes these recurring oscillations within the metabolic day. It modulates when and how long specific physiological states predominate, altering the sequencing of hormonal and substrate signals without redefining their fundamental roles.

Intermittent fasting, viewed mechanistically, is rhythmic modulation within an already rhythmic metabolic system.

Intermittent fasting is often interpreted through visible outcomes rather than structural analysis. Short-term changes are observed, attributed to the most salient variable, and generalized into rule. Several recurring claims illustrate this pattern.

"Fasting causes fat loss."

During fasting intervals, insulin levels decline and lipolysis increases. Fatty acids are mobilized from adipose tissue and oxidized for energy. This shift is measurable. It is also transient. The body increases fat utilization when exogenous energy is absent because it must maintain function. The presence of fat oxidation during a fasting hour does not determine whether net fat mass decreases across weeks.

Body composition reflects cumulative energy balance over time. If total intake across the feeding window equals or exceeds expenditure, fat mass may remain stable or increase despite repeated fasting intervals. If intake falls below expenditure consistently, fat mass may decline whether meals are compressed or dispersed.

One commonly misunderstood mechanism is the difference between fuel selection and fat loss. Fuel selection describes what the body is burning at a given moment. Fat loss describes net change in stored adipose tissue over extended periods. The body may burn more fat during a fasting morning and more carbohydrate during an evening meal. Over twenty-four hours, these shifts can balance out. Without sustained negative energy balance, adipose stores are not obligated to decline.

A second misunderstood mechanism involves glycogen depletion. Extended fasting reduces liver glycogen stores. Because glycogen binds water, early weight reductions may reflect glycogen and associated fluid loss rather than adipose tissue reduction. Visible scale changes reinforce the perception that fasting directly eliminates fat, even when tissue composition has not meaningfully shifted. This initial response can anchor belief before longer-term patterns emerge.

"Intermittent fasting is superior to calorie control."

Comparisons between timing structures and traditional calorie distribution often assume that fasting carries unique metabolic leverage independent of intake. However, when total calories are equated in controlled settings, body composition outcomes are frequently similar across different meal frequencies. Differences that do appear are often mediated by adherence, appetite containment, or behavioral simplification rather than by distinct biochemical pathways exclusive to fasting.

Intermittent fasting can reduce spontaneous intake in some individuals by narrowing eating opportunities. This behavioral containment may produce an energy deficit without explicit calorie counting. The mechanism is indirect. The timing structure modifies opportunity and appetite rhythm, which may influence quantity. Superiority claims conflate the structural tool with the behavioral effect it sometimes produces.

Timing may alter how intake is experienced and distributed. It does not eliminate the requirement that intake and expenditure reconcile over days and weeks.

"Longer fasting is always better."

Duration is often treated as a linear gradient of benefit. If twelve hours without food produces measurable fat oxidation, eighteen hours is presumed superior. If a daily window produces change, alternate-day fasting is presumed more effective. This escalation logic overlooks diminishing returns and compensatory responses.

Prolonged fasting increases time spent in post-absorptive metabolism. It may also increase hunger intensity, reduce spontaneous physical activity, or alter hormonal signals that influence recovery. Beyond certain durations, escalating fasting intervals can shift from manageable metabolic stress to cumulative strain.

Physiological systems adapt to repeated stimuli, but adaptation requires adequate recovery and sufficient energy availability across the cycle. When fasting duration expands without corresponding adjustments elsewhere, the net effect may be increased volatility rather than incremental benefit.

The relationship between fasting duration and outcome is therefore non-linear. Extension does not guarantee proportional advantage.

"More restriction equals more benefit."

Restriction often produces rapid visible change, particularly when prior intake was unstructured. Early momentum reinforces the belief that intensifying constraint will amplify results. Yet increased restriction narrows the margin for recovery and behavioral flexibility. It can heighten preoccupation with food, reduce dietary variety, and create cycles of rigidity followed by compensation.

A behavioral misinterpretation frequently accompanies this pattern: identity attachment. Fasting becomes a marker of discipline or metabolic sophistication. Shorter windows are equated with greater control. Social narratives may frame adherence as evidence of superiority. When identity fuses with structure, evaluation becomes less objective. Escalation may continue not because it improves outcomes, but because it reinforces self-concept.

This dynamic can obscure early warning signals. Fatigue, sleep disruption, or persistent irritability may be reframed as necessary discomfort rather than feedback indicating imbalance. The structure shifts from tool to ideology.

Autophagy and "metabolic reset" claims

Brief references to cellular cleanup processes or metabolic "resets" often

processes or metabolic "resets" often amplify expectations. Autophagy is a continuous cellular recycling process influenced by nutrient availability, energy status, and other signals. While fasting can modulate these pathways, translating acute molecular responses into sweeping claims of system-wide renewal oversimplifies complex regulation. The body does not reset metabolism to a baseline state through isolated fasting intervals. Adaptation reflects cumulative inputs, not singular events.

A structural reason why short-term results are generalized into universal rules lies in temporal compression of observation. Early changes—reduced scale weight, heightened mental clarity, decreased meal frequency—occur within days or weeks. These are salient and immediate. Long-term variables such as adaptive energy expenditure, behavioral sustainability, and tissue composition evolve more slowly. Humans infer causality from visible shifts, particularly when those shifts align with expectations.

Another structural factor is selection bias in anecdotal reporting. Individuals for whom a timing structure produces favorable results are more likely to describe their experience publicly. Those who encounter instability may discontinue quietly. The visible narrative skews toward success, reinforcing the perception of universal applicability.

Misinterpretation often arises when partial mechanisms are isolated from the system in which they operate. Increased fat oxidation during fasting is observed and equated with guaranteed fat loss. Reduced eating opportunities are observed and equated with metabolic superiority. Early weight change is observed and equated with permanent transformation. Each observation contains truth at a narrow scale. Each becomes distortion when extended without context.

Intermittent fasting is frequently evaluated through outcomes detached from structural analysis. When mechanism, duration, behavior, and cumulative balance are considered together, categorical claims lose coherence.

Misinterpretation emerges when partial observation is extended into general rule.

This book examines intermittent fasting as a structural variable within human metabolism. Its focus is not advocacy or opposition, but analysis.

The primary object of examination is timing pattern—how different distributions of feeding intervals reorganize metabolic exposure across days and weeks. Timing patterns influence hormonal sequencing, substrate availability, appetite rhythm, and behavioral containment. These patterns will be considered in relation to adaptive response: how the organism adjusts to repeated exposure to compressed or extended feeding intervals over time.

Hormonal signaling will be addressed not as isolated spikes or single pathways, but as coordinated systems. Insulin, leptin, ghrelin, cortisol, thyroid hormones, and reproductive signaling do not operate independently. Their responses are shaped by cumulative energy availability, sleep integrity, stress exposure, and prior dieting history. Intermittent fasting alters the temporal arrangement in which these signals appear. The interaction between timing and endocrine response requires contextual framing rather than categorical interpretation.

Stress interaction will be treated as part of the metabolic landscape. Feeding compression exists alongside psychological demand, occupational pressure, environmental strain, and physical training load. The body integrates these inputs simultaneously. A timing structure introduced into a low-demand context may be absorbed differently than the same structure applied during periods of high external or internal load. The analysis will therefore consider how timing interacts with cumulative stress exposure rather than treating it as an isolated input.

Recovery integrity forms another structural pillar. Sleep duration and quality, micronutrient sufficiency, total caloric adequacy, and rest from physical exertion all influence how metabolic systems adapt. When recovery bandwidth narrows, tolerance for additional variability may narrow as well. Intermittent fasting does not operate outside these constraints. It functions within them.

Body composition will be discussed within the framework of energy balance and nutrient partitioning. Changes in fat mass and lean mass emerge from sustained relationships between intake, expenditure, hormonal signaling, and mechanical loading. Timing can influence these variables indirectly by shaping appetite, feeding opportunity, and substrate cycling. It does not guarantee fat reduction or muscle preservation in isolation. Partitioning efficiency—how nutrients are allocated toward storage or oxidation—will be examined as context-dependent rather than universally optimized by feeding compression.

Sex-specific differences warrant careful consideration. Hormonal milieu differs between males and females, particularly with respect to reproductive signaling and energy availability thresholds. Women may exhibit greater sensitivity to sustained low energy availability, with downstream effects on menstrual regularity and thyroid function. Men may display different patterns of appetite compensation or hormonal fluctuation under similar timing structures. These distinctions do not imply fragility or superiority; they reflect physiological variation that shapes response.

Aging introduces additional variables. Insulin sensitivity, muscle protein synthesis responsiveness, sleep architecture, and recovery speed often shift across decades. The margin for aggressive energy restriction may narrow as muscle mass preservation becomes more critical for metabolic stability. Feeding timing intersects with these age-related changes in ways that require nuanced evaluation rather than uniform prescription.

Training load and occupational demand further modulate response. Endurance athletes, shift workers, manual laborers, and cognitively demanding professionals experience differing patterns of energy expenditure and recovery requirement. A compressed feeding window during periods of high physical output may influence performance and recovery differently than during sedentary phases. Similarly, irregular work schedules can disrupt circadian alignment, altering how timing structures interact with metabolic rhythm.

Behavioral adherence functions as a systems variable rather than a peripheral concern. Timing patterns may simplify eating decisions for some individuals by reducing grazing and unstructured intake. For others, rigid windows may increase preoccupation with food or social friction. Sustainability depends not only on metabolic tolerance but on psychological integration. A structure that cannot be maintained without escalating strain becomes unstable regardless of its theoretical efficiency.

Intermittent fasting applied briefly may produce different responses than when integrated across months or years. Repetition alters adaptation. The organism does not encounter feeding compression as a single event but as a recurring input layered onto existing patterns. Long-horizon application therefore requires evaluation of cumulative recovery, sustained energy sufficiency, and stability across cycles rather than isolated short-term outcomes. Durability, not immediacy, determines whether a timing structure integrates successfully.

Clear boundaries are necessary.

This book does not prescribe protocols, endorse named formats, promote accelerated fat loss claims, construct escalation hierarchies, or frame performance optimization apart from metabolic context.

Identity-based narratives surrounding fasting—discipline as virtue, deprivation as proof of commitment, superiority through constraint—are outside the scope of this analysis. The focus remains structural and mechanistic rather than ideological.

Intermittent fasting will be evaluated as one variable among many within a dynamic metabolic system, and its implications will be examined in relation to context rather than in isolation.

Intermittent fasting occupies a specific place within the broader landscape of metabolic regulation. It is a tool of arrangement. It alters when energy enters the system, not what the system fundamentally is.

Its effects depend on the structure into which it is introduced and the load it is asked to carry. A timing structure may simplify intake patterns in one context and complicate them in another. It may reduce variability in some environments and introduce it in others. Its role is defined by interaction.

Within metabolic systems, no single variable operates independently. Sleep, activity, psychological demand, hormonal status, food quality, total intake, and social rhythm coexist and overlap. Timing intersects with each of these. It does not replace them. It does not override them. It modifies their sequencing.

For this reason, evaluation requires distance from attachment. When a feeding structure becomes ideological—framed as proof of discipline, identity, or metabolic advantage—analysis narrows. Structural assessment shifts toward defense or advocacy. Stability, however, depends on flexibility and calibration rather than allegiance.

Long-horizon integration offers a different orientation. Rather than treating feeding timing as an intervention to test for immediate transformation, it can be observed as a pattern introduced into an ongoing system. Over time, patterns either integrate smoothly or generate friction. The assessment becomes less about rapid outcome and more about durability.

Amplification is often mistaken for progress. Extending fasting windows, compressing intake further, or intensifying constraint can create visible short-term shifts. Yet stability rarely emerges from continuous amplification.

Decision neutrality supports this long-horizon view. It is an organizational choice that can be adjusted, expanded, reduced, or discontinued without moral weight.

When evaluated structurally, intermittent fasting becomes neither promise nor threat. It is a variable that can be examined, calibrated, and contextualized. Its relevance is determined by how it interacts with sleep patterns, workload, recovery capacity, and energy sufficiency over extended time frames.

Sustainable health does not emerge from intensity alone. It reflects the alignment of multiple inputs within tolerable ranges. Timing participates in that alignment when integrated thoughtfully. When isolated from context or elevated above other variables, it loses proportionality.

The appropriate question is not whether intermittent fasting is inherently effective or inherently flawed. The question is how it fits within the architecture of a given metabolic system across time.

Intermittent fasting is a timing variable within a broader metabolic system and must be evaluated in context rather than adopted by allegiance.

Fasting as a Timing Variable

Fasting can be understood as a structural input into a metabolic system. A structural input is not defined by intensity, effort, or extremity. It is defined by placement and repetition. Within physiology, placement across time determines signal exposure. Repetition determines adaptation. Fasting, viewed through this lens, functions as a regulator of temporal exposure rather than a measure of deprivation.

Timing describes sequencing and interval placement; intensity describes magnitude. A twelve-hour interval and a twenty-hour interval differ in duration, but both are expressions of temporal arrangement. The magnitude of metabolic stress they produce depends on context, not duration alone.

Timing also differs from duration when considered structurally. Duration is a measurement of hours without intake. Timing includes duration, but it also includes frequency and regularity. A single extended fast does not necessarily reorganize a metabolic system. Repeated placement of fasting intervals at consistent points across days becomes a patterned input. The system responds not only to how long the interval lasts, but to how predictably it appears.

Within metabolic regulation, signal exposure across time matters. Hormones are not defined solely by peak levels; they are defined by cumulative exposure. Insulin, cortisol, and other regulators exert influence through repeated oscillation. The length of time tissues are exposed to elevated insulin across days contributes to downstream signaling effects related to nutrient partitioning and storage. Likewise, the length of time spent in lower-insulin, post-absorptive states shapes substrate mobilization patterns and enzymatic expression.

Fasting therefore operates as exposure control. It alters the total hours across a cycle during which certain signals predominate. A feeding pattern distributed across sixteen waking hours produces a different exposure curve than one compressed into eight. The difference is not whether insulin appears, but how long it remains elevated across the week.

When timing patterns repeat, tissues adapt. Enzymatic activity adjusts to recurring substrate availability. Appetite hormones begin to anticipate feeding windows. Peripheral tissues modify sensitivity according to the rhythm of exposure. Adaptation is not immediate. It emerges through cycles.

This is why fasting cannot be reduced to "skipping meals." Skipping a single meal may transiently extend a fasting interval, but without repetition the system has little reason to recalibrate. Structural timing implies consistent arrangement. When fasting intervals occur at similar times across days, metabolic signaling begins to organize around expectation.

Temporal consistency carries implications distinct from variability. A consistent feeding window produces stable anticipation patterns. Ghrelin pulses align. Digestive readiness synchronizes. Glucose handling becomes more predictable. When timing fluctuates widely—late-night intake one day, early intake the next—signal anticipation fragments. The metabolic system can tolerate variability, but repeated irregularity erodes stable anticipation.

Cumulative signaling effects accrue gradually. If feeding windows are consistently compressed, cumulative insulin exposure across the week may decline relative to continuous grazing, assuming total intake remains stable. Conversely, if compression leads to larger, denser meals, peak insulin levels may increase even as total exposure time decreases. These patterns differ not only in magnitude but in contour.

Contour influences tissue response. Muscle and adipose tissue respond to repeated exposure patterns. Periods of lower insulin signaling may permit greater reliance on endogenous fuel between meals. Periods of concentrated feeding may alter nutrient partitioning depending on activity levels and glycogen status. The pattern, not the isolated event, shapes adaptation.

Consider two individuals adopting an identical eight-hour feeding window beginning at noon. Both maintain similar total caloric intake. The first individual maintains stable sleep, moderate activity, and consistent meal composition. Over time, appetite rhythms consolidate around midday and evening. Energy levels stabilize during the morning fasting interval. Body composition remains steady or gradually shifts in alignment with intake.

The second individual maintains the same nominal window but experiences irregular sleep and high occupational stress. Morning fasting coincides with elevated cortisol and reduced sleep duration. Hunger intensifies, and meals within the window become larger and more rapid. Evening intake extends closer to bedtime, fragmenting sleep further. Although the window is identical, cumulative exposure to stress hormones and sleep disruption modifies metabolic response. Outcomes diverge not because of the window itself, but because of the context into which it is inserted.

Timing as a structural input therefore interacts with other temporal variables: sleep cycles, activity rhythms, and stress exposure. The metabolic system integrates these signals simultaneously. Fasting reorganizes one dimension of timing; it does not suspend the others.

An instability pattern can emerge when timing is poorly integrated with daily structure. For example, repeated late-night feeding compression—where the majority of intake occurs in the final hours before sleep—can create overlapping signals. Insulin elevation, digestive activity, and sympathetic arousal may intersect with the body's transition toward nocturnal recovery. Sleep fragmentation may follow. Morning appetite rhythms may become erratic. Over time, the timing structure intended to consolidate intake instead destabilizes circadian coherence.

Such instability does not arise from fasting as an abstract concept. It arises from mismatched signal placement. When the temporal arrangement conflicts with other biological rhythms, cumulative strain can appear.

Distinguishing timing from intensity also prevents escalation logic. Extending fasting duration is not inherently equivalent to improving metabolic regulation. Without regard to exposure contour and contextual fit, longer intervals may simply shift stress load rather than refine adaptation. Structural timing evaluates where signals fall across cycles, not how extreme they appear in isolation.

Fasting as a timing variable is therefore best conceptualized as repeated signal placement across metabolic cycles. Its influence emerges from cumulative exposure patterns and the system's adaptive response to those patterns, not from isolated acts of omission.

A single fasting interval produces an acute response. Repeated fasting intervals produce adaptation.

The distinction is structural. Acute response reflects the body's immediate adjustment to altered nutrient availability. Hormonal shifts occur. Substrate selection changes. Appetite may intensify or diminish temporarily. These reactions are transient and often pronounced during initial exposure. Adaptation, by contrast, reflects recalibration across cycles. It unfolds gradually as tissues adjust enzymatic activity, receptor sensitivity, and anticipatory signaling in response to repeated temporal patterns.

When fasting intervals recur at consistent points across days, metabolic systems begin to anticipate them. Enzymes involved in fatty acid transport and oxidation may increase in activity during predictable post-absorptive periods. Mitochondrial efficiency in handling fatty acids can improve when exposure to these substrates becomes regular rather than sporadic. Glycogen utilization patterns may stabilize as the body adjusts to recurrent depletion and replenishment cycles.

These changes are not instantaneous. Early fasting intervals often feel energetically disruptive because substrate switching is less efficient. The organism may rely more heavily on stress hormones to maintain blood glucose stability. Over repeated cycles, reliance on acute compensatory signaling can diminish as baseline enzymatic pathways adjust. The shift reflects recalibration rather than escalation.

Substrate efficiency shifts are incremental. When repeated fasting intervals lengthen time spent relying on endogenous fuel, tissues may become more efficient at mobilizing and oxidizing fatty acids during those windows. This does not eliminate carbohydrate metabolism. It refines the transition between fuels, reducing volatility in energy availability. The effect depends on consistent exposure and adequate recovery between cycles.

Appetite entrainment follows a similar trajectory. During early exposure to a new feeding window, hunger often appears at previously habitual mealtimes. Over several weeks, ghrelin pulses begin to align with the updated schedule. Hunger becomes more concentrated around expected feeding periods and less intrusive outside them. This entrainment illustrates that appetite rhythm adapts to repetition rather than to isolated deviations.

The novelty effect often obscures this process. Early adoption of a new timing structure can produce noticeable shifts in energy levels, body weight, or perceived mental clarity. Part of this response reflects the disruption of previous patterns—reduced snacking, decreased late-night eating, or increased dietary awareness. As repetition normalizes the pattern, these novelty-driven effects may attenuate. Initial weight reduction related to glycogen depletion or reduced grazing may slow as the system stabilizes around a new equilibrium.

An early response that does not always persist long-term is spontaneous appetite suppression. Some individuals report markedly reduced hunger during the first weeks of compressed feeding. Over time, appetite frequently recalibrates to match total energy needs. Intake within the feeding window may gradually increase to compensate for extended fasting intervals. The initial suppression was transitional, not necessarily a permanent recalibration.

Adaptation requires both repetition and recovery. Repeated fasting intervals act as recurring stimuli. Recovery—adequate energy intake, sleep, and rest—allows systems to adjust without accumulating strain. When repetition occurs without sufficient recovery, the adaptive signal can become destabilizing.

An instability pattern emerges when fasting intervals are repeated during periods of inadequate total intake or compromised sleep. Rather than improving substrate efficiency, the body may downregulate energy expenditure to conserve resources. Resting metabolic rate can decline modestly. Spontaneous physical activity may decrease. Subjective fatigue can increase. These changes represent protective adaptation rather than dysfunction, but they indicate that repetition has exceeded available recovery capacity.

Adaptation also operates within constraints. Systems recalibrate within physiological limits defined by genetics, hormonal milieu, and life stage. For example, individuals with prolonged histories of aggressive dieting may exhibit slower or blunted metabolic flexibility improvements when introducing fasting intervals. Prior adaptation to energy scarcity can narrow the margin for additional stimulus. In such cases, adaptation may plateau sooner than anticipated.

Plateau does not imply failure. It reflects a new steady state under the existing configuration of timing and intake. Once enzymatic pathways, appetite rhythms, and substrate cycling stabilize, further changes require either altered stimulus or altered context. Extending fasting duration beyond this point does not guarantee additional adaptation. The system may redistribute stress rather than recalibrate further.

Another constraint arises when external demands fluctuate. Increased training load, occupational stress, or disrupted sleep can interfere with ongoing adaptation. The same fasting interval that previously integrated smoothly may feel destabilizing under new conditions. Adaptation is not fixed; it remains contingent on the broader environment in which repetition occurs.

The temporal dimension of adaptation also matters. Early weeks often involve perceptible shifts. Subsequent months may reflect quieter stabilization. Long-term integration depends less on acute metabolic responses and more on whether the pattern remains compatible with daily structure. A timing arrangement that can be repeated without escalating strain is more likely to integrate fully than one requiring continuous override of appetite or fatigue cues.

Repeated signal exposure shapes tissue response. Enzymes adjust to predictable substrate patterns. Appetite aligns with expected feeding windows. Energy stability improves as transitions become less abrupt. These adaptations are gradual and contingent, emerging across cycles rather than within single intervals.

Adaptation to fasting timing is therefore not the product of isolated abstention but of repeated, recoverable signal exposure across metabolic cycles.

Timing patterns do not operate in isolation. They exist within broader rhythms that include sleep, activity, occupational demand, and psychological stress. The degree to which a fasting structure integrates smoothly depends not only on its duration but on its consistency and its alignment with these parallel cycles.

Consistent timing provides predictable signal sequencing. When feeding windows open and close at similar points across days, anticipatory mechanisms stabilize. Digestive readiness aligns with expected intake. Appetite signals cluster within defined periods. Energy availability follows a patterned curve. This consistency allows adaptation to consolidate. The organism becomes efficient at transitioning between states because transitions occur within recognizable boundaries.

Irregular timing introduces variability into these transitions. Feeding windows that shift daily—early one day, late the next—alter the sequencing of hunger signals, substrate utilization, and recovery rhythms. While metabolic systems can tolerate occasional deviation, repeated irregularity fragments predictability. Hormonal anticipation may become diffuse rather than concentrated. Sleep timing may drift relative to final food intake. Appetite intensity may fluctuate in less stable patterns.

For example, late-evening intake following extended daytime fasting may overlap with the body's transition toward nocturnal recovery. Digestive activity, elevated insulin, and sympathetic activation may coincide with melatonin release and parasympathetic dominance. The organism receives mixed cues—prepare for recovery while simultaneously processing concentrated intake. Over repeated cycles, this misalignment can alter sleep continuity and morning energy stability.

Similarly, early-morning high-demand training layered onto prolonged fasting may introduce competing signals. Muscular work requires substrate availability. If repeated without sufficient energy integration later in the day, recovery signals may weaken. The timing pattern itself has not changed, but its interaction with increased workload introduces strain.

Adaptation begins to fragment when the cumulative demands of timing, sleep, and workload exceed the organism's capacity for integration. Fragmentation does not always present as dramatic dysfunction. It may appear as subtle increases in hunger volatility, reduced training output, or slower recovery between sessions. Appetite may become less predictable. Sleep onset may lengthen. Energy levels may oscillate more sharply.

Reversal of previously stable adaptation can occur when contextual variables shift. An individual who maintained consistent feeding compression during a period of moderate workload may adapt with stable energy and appetite rhythms. If occupational stress increases or sleep becomes irregular, the same timing pattern may produce heightened fatigue or increased hunger intensity. The adaptation achieved under one set of conditions does not automatically persist under altered demands.

For example, consider an individual who integrated a consistent feeding window while working a stable daytime schedule. Appetite entrained predictably. Energy levels remained steady. Months later, the individual transitions to rotating shift work with variable sleep timing. Feeding windows now intersect unpredictably with sleep episodes. The previously stable adaptation begins to regress. Hunger cues become erratic. Recovery from work-related fatigue slows. The timing structure has not inherently failed; its alignment with the broader rhythm has shifted.

Irregular timing itself can become an instability pattern. Alternating between extended fasting days and unrestricted late-night eating on other days produces wide oscillations in hormonal and behavioral signals. The body alternates between concentrated energy intake and extended deprivation without consistent patterning. Appetite signals may intensify unpredictably. Sleep may vary according to intake timing. The lack of stable placement blunts consolidation of adaptation.

Variability is tolerated within ranges. Occasional deviations—social meals extending later than usual or unexpected schedule changes—do not inherently dismantle adaptation. The organism is resilient to moderate perturbation. Destabilization tends to occur when irregularity becomes the rule rather than the exception. Without repeated alignment, anticipatory mechanisms cannot stabilize, and adaptive gains may diminish.

Adaptive limits are also shaped by life stage and hormonal milieu. In younger individuals with high recovery bandwidth, variability may be absorbed more readily. During phases of hormonal transition—such as perimenopause or periods of reduced sex hormone stability—energy signaling and appetite regulation can become more sensitive to disruption. A timing pattern previously integrated may require recalibration as hormonal context changes.

Metabolic flexibility itself has boundaries. While repeated exposure to fasting intervals can enhance efficiency in substrate transition, this flexibility does not expand indefinitely. Under sustained high demand, such as increased training volume or chronic sleep restriction, flexibility can narrow. Transitions between fuel states may become more abrupt or energetically costly. What once felt stable may begin to require greater effort to maintain.

Repeated misalignment can blunt prior adaptive gains. If sleep disruption accumulates alongside feeding compression, appetite rhythms may desynchronize. If occupational stress increases without adjustment in energy intake timing, recovery signals may weaken. The system responds to the net configuration of inputs, not to timing in isolation.

Metabolic flexibility strengthens under consistent, aligned repetition and weakens when contextual coherence erodes. Duration of fasting alone does not determine adaptive outcome. Placement of that duration within the broader temporal environment exerts equal influence.

Adaptive capacity is shaped by the consistency of timing and its alignment with sleep, workload, and hormonal context, rather than by fasting length alone.

Fasting operates within a multilayered regulatory system. Timing is one layer among several that collectively shape metabolic experience across days and months.

Energy availability forms a foundational layer. Total intake relative to expenditure determines whether tissues are maintained, reduced, or accumulated over time. Feeding windows influence how intake is distributed, but they do not alter the requirement that sufficient energy be present to support basal function, activity, and recovery. When energy availability remains chronically low, the body initiates conservation responses regardless of how precisely intake is timed. Conversely, when intake chronically exceeds expenditure, compression alone does not prevent surplus storage.

Sleep architecture represents another structural layer. Deep sleep supports hormonal regulation, glucose control, appetite balance, and tissue repair. Feeding timing can influence sleep quality depending on placement, but it cannot compensate for persistent sleep restriction. If an individual consistently sleeps five hours per night, narrowing the eating window does not restore the hormonal environment typically supported by seven to eight hours of stable sleep. Timing may refine the daily pattern of intake; it does not reconstruct nocturnal recovery.

Workload, whether physical or cognitive, adds demand. High training volume increases substrate turnover and recovery requirements. Intense cognitive demand elevates sympathetic tone and may alter appetite signaling. In such contexts, feeding compression modifies how energy enters the system, yet it cannot negate the need for adequate fuel and rest. Timing may improve scheduling efficiency, but it cannot offset chronic under-recovery.

Across weeks and months, timing functions as an exposure architecture. It shapes how many hours are spent in fed versus post-absorptive states and how often transitions occur. This contour influences subjective energy stability, appetite rhythm, and substrate cycling. However, it operates within boundaries defined by energy sufficiency, sleep continuity, and workload balance.

Structural adjustment differs from systemic correction. Adjusting feeding windows can reorganize the daily pattern of intake. Systemic correction involves addressing underlying mismatches such as chronic sleep deprivation, sustained caloric deficit, or unmanaged stress load. Timing may coexist with systemic correction, but it does not replace it.

For example, consider an individual experiencing persistent fatigue and slowed recovery due to inadequate total caloric intake relative to training demands. Shifting to a narrower feeding window may initially create a sense of structure and control. Yet if total intake remains insufficient, fatigue will likely persist. The issue lies not in meal distribution but in energy mismatch. Without addressing the underlying deficit, timing modification does not resolve the imbalance.

Similarly, increasing fasting duration does not correct circadian misalignment. If late-night screen exposure and irregular bedtimes fragment sleep, extending the fasting interval into the morning does not restore sleep architecture. It may even amplify morning fatigue if energy intake is delayed while sleep remains compromised. The fundamental constraint resides in disrupted recovery rhythm, not in feeding placement.

Improvements attributed to timing often reflect concurrent pattern shifts. When individuals adopt a structured feeding window, they may simultaneously reduce late-night snacking, improve food quality, or align meals with daylight hours. Sleep may improve as evening eating declines. Reduced grazing may simplify decision-making and lower total intake. These changes are not solely consequences of fasting duration; they are components of a broader behavioral realignment.

Long-term stability depends on proportional alignment across variables. Feeding timing, energy intake, sleep duration, and workload must coexist within tolerable ranges. When one variable is intensified without regard for the others, strain accumulates. When variables align proportionally, adaptation stabilizes.

There are constraints beyond which increasing fasting duration offers diminishing returns. If workload rises sharply without parallel adjustment in intake or recovery, extending fasting intervals adds stress without resolving the mismatch. Likewise, in periods of life characterized by hormonal transition or increased recovery needs, more aggressive timing may narrow flexibility rather than enhance it.

Timing refines distribution; it does not replace foundational biological requirements. It can shape daily metabolic experience by altering signal contour across time. It cannot substitute for adequate sleep, sufficient energy, or balanced workload.

Across extended time frames, proportionality becomes more important than precision. A feeding window maintained for years exerts influence not through extremity but through consistency. If the timing structure integrates without eroding sleep, recovery, or energy sufficiency, its contour becomes part of the system's baseline rhythm. If it repeatedly conflicts with those layers, strain accumulates gradually rather than dramatically. Long-term stability reflects whether timing harmonizes with foundational inputs rather than competing with them.

Fasting as a timing strategy therefore functions as a regulatory contour within the metabolic system—shaping how signals are distributed across cycles while remaining subordinate to the broader constraints that govern energy balance, recovery, and physiological stability.

Across months and years, feeding timing becomes more than a daily decision. It becomes a stable background pattern.

Exposure architecture refers to the cumulative shape of metabolic signaling across extended periods—the contour traced repeatedly over weeks rather than the peak of a single day. How many hours are spent in relative energy abundance. How many hours are spent mobilizing internal reserves. How often transitions occur. How predictable those transitions are. Over time, this contour exerts influence on appetite rhythm, substrate preference, and perceived energy stability.

In this sense, timing functions less as an event and more as a background pattern. The body adapts to repeated contours. If the contour is moderate and consistent, adaptation consolidates quietly. If it is aggressive and frequently altered, adaptation remains provisional.

Contour matters more than extremity because metabolic systems respond to repeated exposure rather than isolated intensity. A severely compressed feeding window practiced intermittently may generate sharp oscillations without allowing stable recalibration. A moderately compressed window practiced consistently may generate smaller oscillations but greater long-term coherence.

Moderate timing frequently integrates more effectively than aggressive compression because it preserves alignment with other physiological demands. For example, a consistent ten-hour feeding window that aligns with daylight hours and supports adequate total intake may integrate with sleep and workload rhythms without requiring compensatory strain. Appetite entrains. Energy remains stable. Recovery remains intact.

By contrast, a four-hour window layered onto a demanding schedule may initially feel efficient but require increasing effort to maintain. Meals become dense. Social flexibility narrows. Sleep timing may shift to accommodate intake. Over time, the contour may create sharper daily contrasts that are harder to sustain within changing life conditions.

The distinction is not "better" versus "worse," but structural coherence versus intensity. Structural coherence exists when timing aligns proportionally with energy needs, sleep patterns, and workload. Intensity refers to how compressed or extended the window appears in isolation. A coherent structure need not be extreme. An extreme structure may lack coherence.

Timing is also calibratable. It is not a fixed identity. Feeding windows can expand or contract in response to shifting demands without abandoning structure altogether. A window that functions well during periods of stable workload may require adjustment during travel, illness, or increased training volume. Calibration preserves adaptability.

Flexibility within structure maintains adaptive capacity. When timing becomes rigid—applied without regard for context—it can narrow the system's ability to respond to new demands. For instance, strict adherence to a narrow evening feeding window during periods of early-morning training may compress recovery and elevate fatigue. Allowing temporal adjustment during such phases preserves alignment without discarding structure entirely.

Rigid adherence can also limit social and environmental integration. When feeding windows cannot accommodate variability in schedule or communal meals, strain accumulates. This strain may not manifest metabolically at first; it may appear behaviorally as preoccupation or friction. Over time, narrowed flexibility can erode sustainability.

Escalation is often mistaken for refinement. Shortening a window from eight hours to six may appear to represent progress. Yet if the original structure was already coherent and integrated, further compression may not improve metabolic stability. It may simply intensify oscillation without proportional gain. Refinement involves alignment and proportionality, not continual narrowing.

Sustainable integration depends on balance among variables. A timing contour that supports adequate intake, aligns with sleep, and accommodates workload can persist across seasons. One that requires constant negotiation with fatigue, hunger volatility, or schedule conflict may prove unstable regardless of its theoretical efficiency.

Over extended periods, the metabolic system reflects the contour to which it has been most consistently exposed. This contour shapes subjective experience—energy, appetite rhythm, perceived stability—as much as it shapes measurable outcomes. Structural timing is not defined by maximal compression, but by coherent integration.

Timing, when viewed architecturally, is an adjustable exposure contour that shapes metabolic experience across cycles without superseding foundational physiological constraints.

Feeding Windows and Energy Distribution

A feeding window does more than determine when eating begins and ends. It determines how energy is distributed within a bounded interval. In this sense, a feeding window functions as distribution architecture.

Distribution architecture refers to how caloric load is arranged across the hours in which intake occurs. Within any given window, energy can be dispersed across multiple meals of moderate size or concentrated into one or two dense episodes. The length of the window establishes duration. Distribution within that window establishes amplitude.

Compression and dispersion are distinct dimensions. Compression refers to how many hours are allocated to intake relative to the day. Dispersion refers to how evenly energy is spread within those hours. A short window can contain evenly spaced, moderate meals. A longer window can still involve highly clustered intake. Window length alone does not determine how energy is experienced physiologically.

Meal density becomes relevant within fixed windows. Dense meals—large caloric loads consumed in brief periods—create sharper hormonal and substrate peaks. Smaller, spaced meals produce lower peaks but extend exposure across more of the window. Total daily exposure may be similar if total intake is unchanged, yet the contour differs significantly.

Distribution therefore modifies the amplitude of signaling, not merely duration. A compressed window with two large meals may reduce the number of postprandial periods but increase the height of each one. A dispersed pattern within the same window may produce more frequent but smaller oscillations. The organism responds to both peak magnitude and cumulative exposure.

The difference between window length and energy concentration is often overlooked. Two individuals may both follow an eight-hour window. One may consume three meals of relatively balanced size spaced across those hours. The other may delay intake until late in the window and consume the majority of daily calories in a single sitting. Both technically adhere to the same window. Their metabolic exposure profiles diverge.

Consider a comparison. Individual A distributes 2,200 calories across three meals at noon, 3 p.m., and 7 p.m., each containing moderate portions. Postprandial responses occur three times, with recovery periods between them. Glycemic excursions remain within predictable ranges. Satiety signals rise and fall in sequence.

Individual B also consumes 2,200 calories between noon and 8 p.m. However, intake is minimal until 6 p.m., followed by a single large meal comprising nearly all daily calories. The feeding window is identical. The distribution is not. The concentrated load produces a pronounced hormonal peak and extended digestive demand within a narrow period. The total exposure time to intake is the same; the amplitude differs.

Clustering intake increases peak load even when total exposure time decreases. A shorter window does not automatically reduce total intake. It may concentrate it. In some cases, compression reduces grazing and lowers cumulative calories. In others, hunger accumulated during fasting leads to rapid and dense consumption once the window opens. The structure of the window does not dictate how energy is partitioned within it.

Hormonal contour across a day reflects this distribution. Concentrated meals create sharper elevations followed by steeper declines. More evenly distributed intake produces gentler oscillations. These differences influence subjective experience—energy stability, satiety duration, and digestive comfort—as well as objective measures such as postprandial glucose variability.

Digestive load is another dimension of distribution architecture. Large, dense meals demand substantial gastric and intestinal processing within a limited time. For some individuals, this load is tolerated without difficulty. For others, concentrated intake may produce bloating, reflux, or prolonged fullness that interferes with subsequent sleep. The feeding window may close, yet digestion continues. Distribution within the window shapes how long physiological processing extends beyond it.

Excessive habitual concentration can polarize appetite regulation. Hunger can intensify sharply before the meal and diminish profoundly afterward, creating pronounced oscillation. Over time, this pattern may increase preoccupation with the feeding event itself. The issue does not arise from window duration alone but from the magnitude of concentration within it.

Appetite regulation also constrains distribution. Satiety signals depend on volume, macronutrient composition, and eating pace. When energy is densely packed into short periods, the rate of ingestion may outpace satiety signaling. Individuals may consume more than intended before fullness registers. Conversely, evenly spaced intake allows satiety cues to recalibrate between meals.

Digestive efficiency places additional limits. The gastrointestinal system can process substantial energy loads, but repeated maximal loads within narrow intervals may alter comfort and meal pacing. When distribution exceeds digestive tolerance, behavioral adjustments often follow—either increased speed to finish within the window or avoidance of certain foods to reduce discomfort. Both further shift the contour.

Window length and distribution interact but remain independent variables. A longer window does not guarantee dispersion; a shorter window does not guarantee concentration. The metabolic system responds to the combined effect of duration and amplitude across days.

Within a defined feeding window, the size of individual meals alters how nutrients are handled in real time. The body processes incoming energy according to both quantity and rate of arrival. When calories are delivered in large, dense meals, the immediate metabolic task differs from that required to handle smaller, spaced portions of the same total intake.

Meal size influences the amplitude of postprandial response. A larger meal introduces a greater glucose load, a greater influx of dietary fat, and a greater total caloric burden at once. The resulting rise in circulating substrates is typically higher and more prolonged than that produced by a smaller meal. The system responds proportionally to the magnitude of the load presented. A moderate meal generates a moderate peak. A large meal generates a larger one.

Amplitude and frequency interact. Fewer meals of greater size reduce the number of postprandial periods but increase the height of each response. More frequent, moderate meals increase the number of responses while lowering the height of each. The total caloric exposure across twenty-four hours may be identical. The pattern of metabolic handling differs.

These differences influence substrate partitioning in the short term. Large meals saturate immediate oxidation pathways more rapidly, increasing the likelihood that excess substrate is directed toward storage during the postprandial period. Smaller meals spaced within the window may allow more complete oxidation of nutrients before the next intake event. This does not eliminate storage; it alters the temporal pattern in which storage and oxidation alternate.

Glycemic volatility illustrates the effect of amplitude. When carbohydrate intake is concentrated into a large meal, blood glucose may rise more sharply and decline more steeply afterward compared to the response to smaller portions. The magnitude of these swings depends on food composition and individual tolerance, but distribution remains a significant factor. Greater peaks are often followed by more pronounced declines. These oscillations can influence perceived steadiness.

Consider two equal-calorie days totaling 2,400 calories within the same eight-hour window. On the first day, intake is divided into three meals of roughly 800 calories each, spaced evenly. On the second day, 1,800 calories are consumed in one meal and the remaining 600 in a smaller earlier meal. Total energy is identical. The metabolic handling differs. The single large meal creates a substantial postprandial load that extends over several hours. The smaller earlier meal produces a modest response. The frequency of exposure decreases; the amplitude increases.

Subjective energy experience often tracks these contours. Moderate, spaced meals may produce smoother energy across the window. A large, concentrated meal may induce a period of pronounced fullness followed by lethargy or a perceptible decline in energy as circulating substrates normalize. These experiences do not necessarily alter long-term tissue change, but they shape day-to-day stability.

Total intake remains the determinant of cumulative tissue balance. Distribution influences how that energy is processed and perceived in the short term.

Satiety sequencing is sensitive to meal size and pacing. Larger meals often require longer digestion time and may produce delayed fullness signals. Satiety hormones and mechanical stretch receptors respond over time. When energy is ingested rapidly in high concentration, intake can exceed satiety cues before they fully register. Smaller meals, especially when eaten at a moderate pace, may allow satiety signaling to align more closely with intake, reducing overshoot within the window.

A constraint emerges when satiety lag intersects with dense intake. If a large portion is consumed quickly to fit within a narrow window, fullness may not arrive until after intake has exceeded intended levels. Repetition of this pattern can increase the risk of habitual overeating within the window, even if fasting intervals are maintained consistently. The feeding window remains intact; distribution within it alters regulation.

An instability pattern related to glycemic volatility can appear when dense, carbohydrate-heavy meals dominate a compressed window. Sharp rises followed by steep declines in blood glucose may produce transient fatigue or heightened hunger later in the window. The subsequent meal may then be consumed in response to perceived energy deficit rather than baseline appetite. This pattern can amplify oscillation within the window, independent of total caloric intake.

Digestive throughput also interacts with distribution. The gastrointestinal system can process large meals, but repeated maximal loads may slow gastric emptying or create prolonged post-meal discomfort. This can alter pacing of subsequent intake or reduce willingness to distribute calories more evenly. Distribution patterns often evolve in response to how the body handles previous loads.

Amplitude and frequency are not opposing strategies but interacting dimensions. Fewer, larger meals increase amplitude and reduce frequency. More, smaller meals increase frequency and reduce amplitude. Within a fixed window, adjusting one inevitably adjusts the other. The organism adapts to both dimensions over time, but subjective experience and short-term metabolic handling are shaped by how these variables are balanced.

Energy stability across the window reflects this balance. When amplitude is moderate and frequency sufficient to prevent extreme oscillation, subjective steadiness often improves. When amplitude becomes excessive relative to digestive and regulatory capacity, oscillation may increase.

Feeding distribution does not override total energy balance. It shapes the contour through which energy is processed within the window. That contour determines the amplitude of metabolic response and the subjective stability experienced across the day.

Energy distribution within a feeding window does not only shape metabolic amplitude; it also shapes appetite rhythm and behavioral regulation. The pattern by which food is arranged across the window influences how hunger is perceived, anticipated, and managed.

Hunger perception is sensitive to both timing and meal structure. When intake is clustered into one or two dense episodes, hunger may intensify sharply prior to those episodes and diminish profoundly afterward. This creates pronounced peaks and valleys in subjective appetite. When intake is spaced more evenly within the window, hunger often rises and falls in smaller oscillations, reducing extremes. The magnitude of perceived hunger is influenced not only by fasting duration but also by how intake is distributed once the window opens.

Anticipatory appetite develops within the boundaries of a fixed window. If meals occur at relatively consistent times inside that window, hunger cues begin to align with those expected intervals. The body learns not only when the window opens, but when within that window food is likely to appear. Structured spacing can create internal predictability. Unstructured grazing inside the window diffuses this predictability.

Grazing differs from structured intake in its cognitive and physiological implications. When energy is consumed in small, continuous amounts throughout the window without defined meal boundaries, appetite signals may never fully resolve. Satiety remains partial, and hunger remains partially active. This pattern can maintain a low-grade preoccupation with food, as intake is frequently considered and negotiated.

Structured intake, by contrast, delineates episodes of eating from periods of non-eating within the window. Clear boundaries can reduce decision frequency. Rather than evaluating whether to eat at each moment of mild hunger, decisions are clustered into defined meal events. For some individuals, this consolidation reduces cognitive load. Decision fatigue may decline when feeding is patterned rather than reactive.

Behavioral containment differs from caloric restriction. Containment refers to the structuring of opportunity and attention, not necessarily to reducing total intake. A feeding window that includes three defined meals may contain grazing behavior without imposing a numerical limit on calories. The individual experiences fewer unplanned eating episodes, even if total intake remains similar. The structure shapes behavior by limiting dispersion of decisions.

One example illustrates this dynamic. An individual previously consumed food intermittently throughout the day—small snacks during work, additional bites in the evening, and late-night intake. After establishing an eight-hour window with three planned meals, grazing episodes decline. Food decisions occur primarily at meal times. Hunger rises in anticipation of those meals and recedes afterward. Total caloric intake may or may not change significantly, but the pattern becomes more consolidated. The distribution structure reduces grazing by providing defined intake points.

However, distribution can also intensify fixation when overly concentrated. If the majority of daily calories are reserved for a single large meal at the end of the window, the hours preceding that meal may become dominated by anticipation. Hunger may build progressively, and attention may narrow toward the upcoming intake. The meal itself can assume disproportionate psychological weight. Repetition of this pattern may increase preoccupation with the feeding event rather than reduce it.

When distribution amplifies scarcity perception within the window, appetite rhythm can polarize. For example, if intake is consistently delayed to the final hour, the earlier portion of the window becomes a prolonged period of waiting. Hunger cues may accumulate rather than oscillate. The eventual meal may be consumed rapidly and in large volume, reinforcing the cycle of buildup and release. Although the feeding window is technically adhered to, the internal rhythm becomes polarized.

Decision fatigue interacts with distribution as well. Continuous grazing requires repeated micro-decisions: whether to eat, what to eat, and how much to eat. These decisions accumulate cognitive load. Structured distribution reduces the number of decision points. Yet excessive rigidity—such as allowing only one meal regardless of hunger variation—can also increase cognitive strain if internal cues conflict with imposed structure.

Social and environmental constraints further shape distribution. Work schedules may limit opportunities for multiple meals within a window. Some occupations allow only one substantial break, leading to concentration of intake by necessity. Social meals often occur in the evening, influencing where energy is clustered. These constraints modify distribution independent of metabolic preference.

A constraint arises when social rhythm consistently conflicts with chosen distribution. If communal dinners occur late but the feeding window closes early, social participation may decline or tension may increase. Alternatively, extending intake to accommodate social rhythm may compress earlier meals, intensifying hunger in the afternoon. Distribution architecture is influenced by external scheduling realities as much as by internal regulation.

Appetite rhythm is not solely physiological; it is shaped by repetition, environment, and expectation. When distribution is coherent with daily structure, hunger tends to become predictable. When distribution conflicts with social or occupational rhythms, unpredictability may increase.

Behavioral containment can stabilize intake patterns by reducing unstructured grazing and consolidating decisions. Over-concentration, however, can elevate fixation by amplifying anticipation and compressing satisfaction into narrow episodes. The effect depends on how distribution interacts with appetite rhythm and daily context.

Within a feeding window, energy distribution acts as a regulator of appetite sequencing and cognitive load, shaping how hunger is experienced and how feeding decisions are organized rather than merely determining how many calories are consumed.

A feeding window can remain intact while internal dynamics fluctuate sharply. The external boundary—when eating begins and ends—may appear consistent. Within that boundary, distribution patterns can generate volatility.

Energy swings often originate from concentrated intake. When a substantial proportion of daily calories is delivered in a single meal, the post-meal period may be marked by pronounced fullness followed by a perceptible decline in energy as circulating substrates are cleared. The intensity of this rise-and-fall sequence depends on meal size, composition, and individual tolerance. Repeated daily, it creates a predictable oscillation inside the window.

For example, an individual who consumes a minimal midday meal followed by a large early-afternoon meal may experience a surge of energy immediately afterward, then recurrent mid-afternoon fatigue several hours later. The window remains open; no fasting rule has been violated. Yet the internal amplitude of intake produces a pattern of daily lethargy aligned with the timing of the concentrated meal. The volatility arises from distribution rather than window duration.

Digestive load compounds this effect. Large, dense meals require sustained gastric and intestinal processing. Blood flow is directed toward digestion. Mechanical fullness can persist for hours. If similar loads are presented daily without variation, recovery between meals may feel incomplete. The next intake event may occur while residual fullness or delayed digestion lingers, narrowing perceptual appetite cues and altering pacing. Over time, repeated overload can create a rhythm of heaviness followed by rebound hunger.

Compensatory intake within the window introduces another form of instability. If early meals are small or delayed, hunger may intensify progressively. Once intake begins in earnest, consumption may accelerate. The latter portion of the window can then become disproportionately large in both quantity and density. The day's caloric total may still fall within the intended range, but internal sequencing becomes skewed toward accumulation at the end.

This pattern often repeats because hunger accumulated earlier in the window primes later intake. Repetition amplifies the oscillation. Early restraint followed by late concentration becomes the default contour. The feeding window remains structurally consistent; amplitude within it becomes polarized.

An instability pattern emerges when late-window overeating becomes compensatory rather than intentional. Intake may extend close to the closing boundary of the window, with larger portions consumed quickly. Satiety lag—where fullness signals trail behind intake—can increase the likelihood of overshoot. Repetition reinforces the cycle: restrained early intake, escalating hunger, dense late intake, and post-meal heaviness.

Distribution can also mask chronic underfeeding. If total caloric intake is low relative to expenditure, yet meals are large and dense within the window, immediate postprandial fullness may obscure the broader deficit. The individual feels physically full during eating episodes, leading to the perception that intake is sufficient. Outside the window, however, energy levels may gradually decline. Subtle fatigue or reduced spontaneous activity can accumulate across days. The window boundary remains stable; internal energy balance does not.

This hidden strain arises because amplitude can create short-term sensory reassurance. A dense meal generates fullness. Fullness does not guarantee sufficiency. When low total intake is packaged into concentrated episodes, the contrast between intense feeding and extended non-feeding may conceal cumulative deficit.

Structural adherence refers to consistent opening and closing times. Internal stability refers to the coherence of energy, digestion, and appetite within those times. It is possible to maintain precise time boundaries while experiencing daily swings in energy and hunger that undermine steadiness.

Instability driven by amplitude is not always immediately visible. It may appear as predictable fatigue at certain hours, variable appetite intensity from day to day, or subtle digestive discomfort that becomes normalized. Because the window itself appears orderly, attention may not turn to distribution as the source of volatility.

Repetition amplifies these patterns. A single day of concentrated intake may produce transient heaviness without consequence. When concentration recurs daily, oscillations become embedded. The body anticipates the surge-and-decline sequence. Appetite may adjust in response to expected scarcity earlier in the window and expected abundance later. This embedded volatility can become self-reinforcing.

Constraints emerge when dense meals coincide with low total intake. Large meals require significant digestive and metabolic handling. If the overall energy provided remains insufficient for workload, the system oscillates between intense post-meal processing and extended low-energy periods. The amplitude is high; the baseline is low. Over weeks, this combination can create cumulative fatigue without obvious deviation from window rules.

The key distinction lies between visible structure and internal coherence. A feeding window can be executed consistently while internal distribution generates pronounced peaks and troughs. Stability is not guaranteed by adherence to time boundaries alone. It depends on how energy is arranged within those boundaries and how that arrangement interacts with daily demands.

Feeding window stability therefore depends on internal distribution coherence rather than simple adherence to temporal limits.

Energy distribution within a feeding window is not a fixed prescription. It is an adjustable contour that can be calibrated without altering the external boundaries of the window itself.

Window length and internal distribution operate as independent but interacting variables. The opening and closing times define duration. The pattern of meals within that duration defines contour. Adjusting contour does not require expanding or compressing the window. It requires altering how energy is arranged inside it.

Moderate dispersion often smooths internal amplitude without extending duration. When intake is divided into two or three proportionate meals rather than concentrated into a single dense episode, post-meal fluctuations tend to become less extreme. Total caloric exposure across the day remains constant. The window remains constant. What changes is the pacing and proportion of delivery.

For example, an individual consuming 2,200 calories within a six-hour window may initially place nearly all intake into one large evening meal. Energy spikes and declines may follow a predictable pattern. Without changing the window or total intake, shifting to two moderate meals spaced evenly within the same six hours can alter the contour. Fullness becomes less abrupt. Energy may feel steadier. Duration of exposure remains identical. Distribution has been refined.

Distribution refinement differs from escalation. Escalation involves intensifying compression or increasing restriction. Refinement involves aligning internal structure with daily demand. Refinement may include redistributing calories more evenly, adjusting meal size to coincide with activity, or shifting intake earlier within the window to support sleep. These changes do not necessarily reduce calories or narrow duration. They reshape contour.

Proportionality between meal size, workload, and sleep is central to this calibration. Larger meals may integrate more smoothly on days with greater physical demand. Smaller, earlier meals may better support evenings intended for rest. Distribution can reflect the energy needs of the day without abandoning the window framework.

Over time, distribution may evolve in response to life phase. During periods of increased training volume, additional moderate meals within the window may support recovery. During phases of lower demand, fewer meals may feel sufficient. Aging, hormonal transition, and occupational shifts may also influence how dense or dispersed intake feels sustainable. Adjusting distribution within a consistent window preserves structural continuity while allowing metabolic flexibility.

Rigid clustering can narrow adaptability. If all intake is habitually reserved for a single event regardless of changing demands, the system may have limited room to adjust. Social obligations, travel, or workload variation may conflict with such rigidity. When distribution cannot flex within the window, strain may accumulate even if the window itself remains stable.

Adjustment preserves flexibility by maintaining alignment between intake contour and daily context. Flexibility does not require abandoning structure. It requires recognizing that structure includes both boundaries and internal arrangement. By recalibrating distribution rather than escalating compression, the feeding window can remain coherent across changing conditions.

Over longer horizons, distribution calibration exerts quiet influence. Small internal adjustments—slightly earlier first meals, modestly reduced density at the final meal, more even spacing across the window—accumulate across months. Because these shifts do not alter total intake or duration, they often escape notice as "change." Yet repeated smoothing of internal oscillations can reduce cumulative volatility.

Exact calorie partitioning at each meal is less consequential than maintaining proportional alignment between intake, activity, and recovery. When distribution approximates demand with reasonable consistency, metabolic handling tends to feel steadier. Minor day-to-day variation does not disrupt this stability as long as the overall contour remains coherent.

Refinement at this level reduces volatility without modifying duration. The window can remain fixed while internal pacing becomes more balanced. A slightly smaller final meal may support more stable sleep.

A modest redistribution toward earlier hours may reduce late-window intensity. These adjustments operate within the same temporal boundary yet alter experiential texture.

Rigid optimization differs from adaptive proportion. Optimization pursues idealized precision—specific gram targets at specific times—often narrowing flexibility. Adaptive proportion emphasizes alignment without rigidity. It accepts that workload, appetite, and social context fluctuate. Distribution becomes responsive rather than fixed, preserving structural integrity while accommodating change.

Over extended periods, proportional calibration allows the feeding window to remain stable without generating internal friction. Distribution then functions not as a rigid rule but as an adjustable contour that maintains alignment between energy flow and lived rhythm.

Energy distribution, when treated as proportional alignment within temporal boundaries, becomes an architectural element that shapes metabolic steadiness across cycles without demanding rigidity or escalation.

The Oscillation Envelope Model

Biological systems do not operate in straight lines. They oscillate.

Feeding and fasting represent alternating phases of energy influx and energy mobilization. Training and recovery represent alternating phases of stress and restoration. Wakefulness and sleep represent alternating phases of expenditure and repair. Stability does not require eliminating oscillation. It requires keeping oscillation within recoverable bounds.

The Oscillation Envelope Model describes the relationship between oscillation amplitude, recovery density, and adaptive bandwidth across time.

Every adaptive system operates within an envelope—a functional range inside which stress and restoration can alternate without long-horizon compression. When oscillation amplitude remains within this envelope, the system maintains coherence. When amplitude repeatedly exceeds the envelope, compression accumulates. The boundary is not moral; it is mechanical.

Imagine a simple graph.

The horizontal axis represents time.

The vertical axis represents metabolic amplitude—the distance between fed and fasted states, between exertion and recovery, between depletion and restoration.

Within this space sits an upper boundary and a lower boundary. These boundaries define adaptive bandwidth.

Between them moves a wave. The wave represents oscillation—the normal rise and fall of biological states. Feeding raises amplitude. Fasting lowers it. Training raises demand. Sleep restores capacity. The wave is not the problem. The boundaries determine stability.

When oscillation amplitude remains comfortably within the envelope, recovery completes before the next stress cycle begins. The system resets fully. Signal coherence is preserved. Appetite remains interpretable. Sleep remains consolidated. Performance ceiling remains intact.

When oscillation amplitude repeatedly approaches or exceeds the boundaries, recovery becomes incomplete. The next stress cycle begins before restoration has resolved. Small deficits accumulate. The envelope does not collapse immediately; it narrows.

Compression is rarely dramatic. It presents as subtle plateau, extended soreness, appetite volatility, light sleep, or a reduced training ceiling. These are not failures of willpower. They are indicators that oscillation amplitude has exceeded recoverable bandwidth relative to context.

Three primary conditions produce envelope compression:

Excess Amplitude

Oscillation depth exceeds recovery capacity. Feeding windows compress too tightly relative to total load. Training intensity escalates without proportional restoration. The wave grows taller than the envelope permits.

Insufficient Restoration Density

Amplitude remains moderate, but sleep fragmentation, stress density, or workload reduce restoration quality. The envelope shrinks while the wave remains unchanged.

Bandwidth Narrowing Without Recalibration

Life phase shifts alter recovery kinetics, hormonal amplitude, or stress-buffering capacity. The envelope gradually narrows across months or years. If structure remains fixed while bandwidth contracts, oscillation begins to press against its boundaries.

The envelope is dynamic. It expands when recovery density increases and stress load moderates. It narrows when stress accumulates, sleep fragments, or total demand rises. It is influenced by body composition, training history, hormonal environment, and life phase. It is not static.

Intermittent fasting operates inside this model as one variable affecting oscillation amplitude. A moderate feeding window may create oscillation that fits cleanly within the envelope. Further compression increases amplitude depth. Whether that increased depth remains adaptive depends on recovery density and bandwidth width, not on discipline or identity.

Escalation often misinterprets plateau as insufficient amplitude. The window tightens. The wave deepens. If bandwidth is unchanged or narrowing, compression increases. The structure appears stronger; the envelope contracts.

Neutrality protects the envelope because neutrality permits recalibration. When structure is treated as adjustable architecture rather than ideological commitment, oscillation amplitude can be modified to match bandwidth shifts. The envelope remains intact because rigidity does not amplify asymmetry.

The objective is not maximal amplitude. It is sustainable oscillation within recoverable bounds.

Oscillation that fits within the envelope produces stability across seasons. Oscillation that repeatedly exceeds it produces compression, even if short-term signals appear productive.

The Oscillation Envelope Model therefore reframes intermittent fasting from a question of intensity to a question of proportional alignment. The clock does not determine outcome. The relationship between amplitude and recovery capacity does.

Intermittent fasting is neutral within the envelope. It becomes compressive only when oscillation amplitude exceeds recoverable bandwidth relative to cumulative load.

Insulin Exposure Across Time

Insulin is often framed as an acute reaction to a meal. It rises in response to incoming nutrients, facilitates glucose uptake and storage, and then declines. Presented this way, attention gravitates toward peak height—how high insulin rises after eating. Yet insulin functions not only as a peak signal but as a temporal exposure curve.

A temporal exposure curve reflects how long, how often, and how repeatedly insulin remains elevated across hours and days. The body responds not merely to isolated peaks, but to cumulative exposure—the integrated presence of the signal over repeated cycles. Elevation itself is normal and necessary. Architecture emerges from repetition.

In this chapter, "insulin exposure" refers to circulating insulin levels across time, shaped by secretion, clearance, tissue sensitivity, and meal distribution. Insulin elevation enables glucose uptake into muscle and adipose tissue, supports glycogen storage, and coordinates nutrient partitioning. The presence of insulin is not pathological. The question is not whether it rises, but how its elevation is patterned.

Duration and frequency define exposure contour. Frequent small meals generate modest elevations that occur repeatedly across the day. Larger, clustered meals produce higher peaks but fewer episodes. In both scenarios, cumulative exposure—the area under the curve—determines total signal presence across time.

"Area under the curve" refers to total integrated exposure. It represents how much insulin is present and for how long, not merely how high it rises at any single moment.

A grazing pattern may sustain moderate insulin levels across most waking hours. A two-meal pattern may produce shorter, higher peaks followed by longer return intervals toward baseline. Caloric totals may be equivalent. The contour differs.

Prolonged moderate elevation maintains tissues in storage-oriented signaling for extended periods. Shorter, higher peaks separated by clearer descent create sharper transitions between fed and post-absorptive states. Neither configuration is inherently pathological. Each represents a different rhythm of exposure.

Repeated exposure shapes adaptation. Biological systems adjust to persistent signaling. If insulin remains elevated across long portions of the day over months or years, tissues may gradually reduce responsiveness—not because insulin is harmful, but because constant signaling diminishes contrast. Clear oscillation preserves dynamic range.

Flattened oscillation occurs when elevation persists with limited descent. Substrate switching—the transition between carbohydrate and fat utilization—may become less distinct. Short-term energy may feel steady. Over time, metabolic flexibility can narrow.

Clearance kinetics shape exposure contour as much as secretion. Rapid descent after a meal restores baseline contrast. Slower descent compresses recovery intervals. When a new meal begins before prior insulin levels have substantially declined, signal stacking can occur. Repeated stacking across days can raise effective baseline exposure.

Return toward baseline is not incidental; it represents a functional reset. Periods near the signal floor allow tissues to resensitize and restore contrast. Without sufficient descent time, oscillatory amplitude narrows.

Circadian alignment influences this process. Insulin sensitivity and clearance often vary across the day. Late meals may descend more slowly than earlier ones. Sleep disruption can further impair next-day clearance. Thus exposure contour reflects not only meal frequency and size, but also timing relative to circadian rhythm and sleep integrity.

Muscle mass significantly influences disposal capacity. Skeletal muscle is a primary site of glucose uptake. Greater muscle mass and regular contraction increase clearance efficiency. Reduced muscle mass narrows disposal capacity. Aging frequently involves incremental shifts in both muscle mass and clearance dynamics, subtly altering exposure contour across years rather than abruptly.

Insulin exposure therefore emerges from multiple interacting variables: meal distribution, total intake, tissue sensitivity, muscle mass, sleep quality, circadian coordination, and life phase. The hormone itself remains consistent. The architecture through which it moves changes.

Long-horizon repetition determines metabolic architecture. A single high peak does not define trajectory. Persistent contour does. Slightly prolonged evening elevations repeated nightly may gradually compress baseline across months. Conversely, modest improvements in clearance—through resistance training, sleep restoration, or improved distribution—may widen oscillatory range when sustained.

Viewing insulin architecturally shifts emphasis from isolated events to repeated patterning. Peaks matter. Descent matters. Baseline matters. Their relationship across time matters more.

Insulin exposure, understood as a temporal structure rather than a moral signal, becomes a question of rhythm and proportion. It is shaped less by a single meal and more by the cumulative sequencing of meals, sleep, activity, and recovery across cycles.

Insulin regulation is defined not only by how high the signal rises, but by how completely it returns toward baseline between elevations. Baseline represents the signal floor—the relative resting level from which each new postprandial rise begins. It is neither zero nor identical across individuals. It reflects underlying metabolic state.

Baseline functions as a reset point. When insulin returns near this floor after a meal, tissues re-enter a state in which substrate mobilization and sensitivity recalibrate. The decline phase is not merely passive. It is an integral component of oscillation. Without sufficient time near baseline, contrast diminishes.

Clearance dynamics determine how quickly insulin declines following elevation. Clearance reflects hepatic extraction, peripheral uptake, receptor responsiveness, muscle mass, activity level, sleep integrity, and prior exposure patterns. Two individuals consuming identical meals may exhibit different descent curves: one returning near baseline within hours, another remaining moderately elevated for longer.

The distinction between a high peak with rapid clearance and a moderate peak with prolonged elevation is structurally meaningful. A high but brief peak may preserve longer baseline intervals. A moderate but sustained elevation compresses baseline time. Cumulative exposure increases when descent is delayed, even if peak magnitude is lower.

Meal timing interacts directly with clearance. When a subsequent meal is consumed before prior elevation has resolved, signals stack. Signal stacking refers to a new elevation layered onto an incompletely cleared baseline. The curve begins from an elevated starting point rather than from the signal floor. Across a day, repeated stacking can progressively elevate effective baseline.

Consider a day structured around mid-morning, early afternoon, and late afternoon intake. If each meal occurs before insulin has substantially declined from the previous one, afternoon baseline may sit above morning levels. The final meal then begins from a higher starting point, further compressing decline before sleep. Cumulative exposure extends not because of extreme peaks, but because return intervals shorten.

An instability pattern can emerge when return-to-baseline intervals remain chronically abbreviated. If intake occurs across most waking hours and clearance is modest, the body may spend minimal time near the signal floor. Oscillatory rhythm flattens. Over weeks, tissue responsiveness may shift—not from isolated peaks, but from sustained exposure with limited recovery between them.

Circadian rhythm further influences clearance. Insulin sensitivity often varies across the biological day. Clearance may be more efficient earlier and slower later, though individual patterns differ. When larger meals occur late, decline may extend into early sleep. Sleep itself shapes regulatory dynamics. Fragmented or shortened sleep can blunt clearance efficiency the following day. Meal timing relative to circadian phase therefore influences both ascent and descent.

Reduced insulin sensitivity constrains clearance. When tissues require greater insulin concentration to achieve comparable glucose uptake, elevation may persist longer. Baseline may remain modestly elevated between meals. In such cases, even moderate meal frequency can produce extended cumulative exposure because descent slows.

Signal stacking becomes more likely when sensitivity is reduced because return intervals lengthen inherently. A spacing pattern that once permitted near-baseline restoration may no longer suffice if clearance slows. Exposure contour reflects both behavior and physiological state.

Baseline is not simply the absence of stimulation. It represents a functional phase of metabolic regulation. During periods near baseline, counter-regulatory processes operate with less opposition. Substrate mobilization proceeds more readily. Sensitivity may recalibrate. When baseline time contracts persistently, oscillatory range narrows.

Insulin elevation itself is not pathological. Elevation enables nutrient storage and repair. The regulatory issue arises not from peaks, but from insufficient descent. Oscillation requires both ascent and return. Without return, exposure accumulates differently.

The distinction between high peak and prolonged moderate elevation becomes clearer within this framework. A substantial meal followed by full decline may preserve broad oscillation. Multiple moderate meals spaced too closely may reduce oscillatory contrast despite lower peaks. Exposure contour cannot be inferred from magnitude alone.

Across days and weeks, patterns of clearance and return shape regulatory adaptation. Consistent opportunity to approach baseline maintains dynamic range. Repeated stacking compresses it. The system adapts to the contour it encounters most consistently.

Return-to-baseline, therefore, is not incidental. It is a structural component of metabolic oscillation and exposure regulation, ensuring that insulin's role as a time-based signal includes both elevation and descent within daily contour.

Metabolic regulation depends not only on signal magnitude or duration, but on rhythm. Insulin operates within an oscillatory pattern—rising with intake, declining between meals, and repeating across days. This oscillation functions as informational signaling. It communicates to tissues when exogenous energy is abundant and when endogenous stores should predominate.

Oscillation creates contrast. Elevation marks a fed state in which nutrient storage and distribution are prioritized. Descent toward baseline marks a shift toward mobilization and internal substrate utilization. The transition between these states is not binary. It unfolds along a gradient. The repetition of that gradient across days trains the system to move between states efficiently.

Metabolic flexibility refers to the capacity to transition between primary fuel sources without excessive volatility in energy availability or physiological strain. Insulin oscillation supports this flexibility by repeatedly exposing tissues to alternating conditions. During elevation, glucose uptake pathways are emphasized. During descent, fatty acid mobilization and oxidation increase. The alternation maintains responsiveness.

Transition carries cost. Shifting from carbohydrate-dominant oxidation to greater reliance on fatty acids requires coordinated enzymatic adjustment and substrate redistribution. When oscillation is consistent and recoverable, this transition cost declines over time. The body becomes more efficient at switching because the switch occurs predictably and repeatedly.

Rhythmic exposure differs structurally from chronic elevation. Chronic elevation compresses oscillatory contrast. If insulin remains modestly elevated for prolonged portions of the day with limited descent, the signal to transition weakens. Substrate switching becomes less distinct. The system remains biased toward fed-state handling for extended intervals.

Consider two patterns. In the first, insulin rises clearly with meals and returns near baseline between them, creating distinct phases of elevation and descent. Over weeks, tissues repeatedly encounter both conditions. Transition becomes fluid. In the second pattern, insulin rarely declines fully due to frequent intake or prolonged clearance. Elevation persists at moderate levels across most waking hours. Oscillatory range narrows. The signal for mobilization becomes less distinct. Transition capacity may diminish gradually because the system is less frequently required to switch.

Flattened oscillation does not imply absence of fluctuation. It implies reduced contrast between peak and baseline and shortened time near the signal floor. Without sufficient contrast, regulatory pathways associated with mobilization may be underutilized. Flexibility depends on repeated exposure to both sides of oscillation.

Dynamic range can be understood as regulatory bandwidth—the span between meaningful elevation and meaningful return. A wide bandwidth allows tissues to interpret when to store and when to mobilize clearly. A narrow bandwidth compresses that distinction. When oscillatory contrast is distinct and repeatable, receptor responsiveness remains calibrated to variation. Cells experience alternating signals with sufficient separation to preserve sensitivity to change.

Repeated cycles of elevation and descent also prime enzymatic pathways. During fed phases, transporters and storage pathways are engaged. During descent, mobilization and oxidative pathways are recruited. Repetition reinforces readiness in both directions. Enzymes are maintained through recurring use across states.

Systems exposed predominantly to one dominant condition—persistent elevation or persistent scarcity—gradually reduce efficiency in the less-utilized direction. If storage-oriented signaling dominates most of the day, mobilization pathways may become comparatively underused. If mobilization dominates due to prolonged underfeeding, anabolic responsiveness may diminish. Switching efficiency depends on rehearsal.

Muted oscillation differs from exaggerated oscillation. Muted oscillation compresses contrast, keeping signals within a narrow band. Exaggerated oscillation produces extreme peaks and troughs that may strain transition capacity. In both cases, dynamic range is compromised—either by flattening or by destabilizing amplitude beyond recoverable limits. Functional flexibility depends on contrast that is distinct yet proportionate.

Metabolic flexibility is therefore sustained not by minimizing oscillation nor by amplifying it excessively, but by maintaining sufficient regulatory bandwidth for repeated, recoverable transition. Insulin oscillation functions as a core mechanism supporting metabolic flexibility through structured cycles of elevation and descent.

Amplitude alone does not define oscillation quality. High peaks with incomplete descent also narrow flexibility if recovery phases are truncated. Conversely, moderate peaks followed by clear descent can preserve rhythmic integrity. The critical variable is recoverable transition.

An instability pattern emerges when oscillation narrows persistently. If exposure remains elevated for most of the day and clearance is slow, tissues may become less responsive to insulin over time. Elevated baseline and blunted peaks reduce dynamic range. Substrate switching becomes less efficient. Energy may feel stable in the short term because transitions are muted, but adaptability declines.

Prolonged underfeeding introduces a different constraint. When total energy intake remains chronically low, oscillation may still occur, but amplitude may diminish due to reduced meal size and lower circulating substrate. The system may remain biased toward mobilization without sufficient refeeding to restore glycogen and anabolic signaling fully. Over time, this can also narrow flexibility, as transitions become one-sided. Oscillation requires both ascent and descent to maintain balance.

Chronic psychological or physiological strain can further influence oscillatory dynamics by altering clearance and sensitivity. When background demands remain elevated, recovery between oscillations may be incomplete. The contour shifts subtly, even if meal timing appears consistent. Flexibility depends not only on oscillation presence, but on the capacity to complete each cycle.

Oscillation functions as more than metabolic fluctuation. It is a regulatory rhythm that preserves responsiveness by alternating conditions. Repeated, recoverable transitions reinforce enzymatic readiness and substrate agility. Flattened exposure—whether from persistent elevation or insufficient refeeding—reduces dynamic range.

Metabolic flexibility is not a static trait. It is a product of repeated oscillatory experience. It strengthens when elevation and descent are distinct and recoverable. It narrows when oscillation compresses or becomes chronically one-sided.

Insulin oscillation functions as a central mechanism supporting metabolic flexibility through repeated, recoverable transitions between fed and post-absorptive states across cycles.

Insulin exposure does not unfold in isolation. Its contour across days reflects not only meal timing and distribution, but also the broader physiological environment in which it occurs. Sleep integrity, circadian alignment, physical training load, muscle mass, aging, and hormonal context each influence how elevations are generated, cleared, and integrated.

Sleep integrity alters exposure contour in subtle but measurable ways. Shortened or fragmented sleep can reduce insulin sensitivity the following day, extending the duration of postprandial elevation. Clearance slows. Baseline may remain modestly elevated between meals. Even when meal timing remains unchanged, the exposure curve shifts because the system's handling capacity is impaired. Over repeated nights of insufficient sleep, this alteration can accumulate, broadening cumulative exposure without modification of intake pattern.

An instability pattern may emerge when sleep disruption becomes habitual. Late-evening intake combined with shortened sleep may produce prolonged overnight elevation and incomplete morning normalization. The next day begins from a higher signal floor. Repetition compresses return intervals and narrows oscillatory range. Feeding pattern may remain constant; clearance context changes.

Circadian alignment further shapes exposure handling. Insulin sensitivity often varies across the biological day, influenced by central and peripheral clocks. Meals consumed during phases associated with reduced sensitivity may produce longer elevations than identical meals consumed during more receptive phases. Thus, identical distribution architecture can generate different exposure contours depending on alignment with internal timekeeping. Circadian misalignment—such as shift work or irregular sleep schedules—can flatten daily oscillatory contrast by impairing coordinated clearance.

Peripheral clocks in liver and skeletal muscle coordinate nutrient handling across the day. These tissue-level clocks regulate expression of enzymes involved in glucose uptake, glycogen synthesis, and substrate oxidation. When feeding patterns align consistently with circadian cues, peripheral clocks synchronize with central timekeeping, supporting predictable clearance and oscillation. When disruption becomes chronic, peripheral clocks may desynchronize. The result is not a change in insulin's function, but a shift in how efficiently tissues respond at given times. Identical intake patterns may therefore generate broader or flatter exposure contours under disrupted circadian coordination.

Muscle contraction functions as a temporal modifier of insulin exposure. During and after contraction, glucose uptake into muscle increases through insulin-dependent and insulin-independent pathways. This can shorten exposure duration by accelerating substrate disposal. Regular contraction across weeks enhances disposal capacity, reinforcing oscillatory contrast. Reduced contraction narrows this capacity.

Sarcopenia—the gradual loss of muscle mass with aging—further constrains disposal bandwidth. With less contractile tissue available, identical elevations may persist longer because the primary reservoir for uptake has diminished. Aging typically compresses oscillatory tolerance gradually rather than abruptly. Clearance may slow incrementally. Sensitivity may decline modestly. Baseline may drift slightly upward. These shifts accumulate across years, narrowing dynamic range without eliminating oscillation entirely.

Hormonal context also influences exposure architecture. Sex hormones, thyroid function, and stress hormones alter insulin sensitivity and clearance efficiency. Changes across menstrual cycles, perimenopause, menopause, and andropause may subtly reshape exposure contour without changes in feeding structure. The signal remains consistent; the responsiveness of tissues evolves.

Physical training load interacts with insulin dynamics. Resistance training increases muscle mass and disposal capacity. Endurance training enhances oxidative efficiency. Excessive training without sufficient recovery, however, may elevate stress signaling and blunt sensitivity. Thus workload and recovery density co-author exposure contour alongside meal distribution.

Context reshapes contour without altering insulin's regulatory purpose. Elevation continues to direct nutrient distribution. Descent continues to permit transition. The difference lies in how efficiently these phases unfold within a given physiological landscape.

Consider two individuals following identical meal timing and distribution. One is well-rested, resistance-trained, and maintains substantial muscle mass with stable circadian rhythm. The other is sleep-deprived, sedentary, and experiences irregular sleep timing with reduced muscle mass. Despite identical feeding architecture, their exposure curves differ. The first may clear elevations efficiently and maintain distinct oscillatory contrast. The second may experience prolonged elevation, elevated baseline, and compressed return intervals. The divergence arises from context, not timing alone.

Constraints accumulate when multiple variables converge. Reduced muscle mass combined with age-related sensitivity shifts may lengthen exposure even under moderate meal patterns. Layered sleep disruption can further slow clearance. The contour broadens not because peaks are excessive, but because descent becomes incomplete.

Insulin exposure therefore functions as a context-dependent regulatory signal. Its impact depends on the organism's capacity to generate clear oscillations and efficient clearance within the broader environment of sleep quality, circadian rhythm, physical activity, muscle mass, age, and hormonal milieu.

Insulin exposure becomes meaningful when viewed across repetition. A single day of altered intake does not define metabolic direction. Regulation is shaped by dominant contour experienced across weeks and months. The body adapts to what recurs.

Exposure functions as accumulated signal memory. Each day contributes to a broader pattern—how long elevations persist, how fully descent occurs, how distinct oscillation remains. Over time, tissues register prevailing rhythm. Sensitivity adjusts. Clearance adapts. Baseline stabilizes relative to that rhythm. The system responds to consistent pattern, not isolated spikes.

Small differences in daily contour compound. Slightly prolonged evening elevation repeated nightly may gradually compress baseline intervals across months. Modestly improved clearance capacity sustained through consistent activity may widen oscillatory range. These changes are rarely dramatic in a single day. They accrue through repetition.

Long-horizon integration therefore outweighs isolated peaks. A pronounced elevation during one meal does not determine metabolic trajectory if descent and recovery follow predictably. Conversely, modest but persistent elevation across most days can reshape exposure architecture over time. Cumulative curve, not exceptional event, guides adaptation.

Distinguishing short-term reaction from long-term architecture clarifies perspective. Acute responses are visible within hours. Architectural shifts unfold across seasons. The regulatory system adjusts to contour encountered most consistently. When oscillation remains clear and recoverable, dynamic range tends to be preserved. When elevation extends and clearance is repeatedly delayed, architecture shifts gradually.

Insulin remains a regulatory hormone within this structure. It coordinates nutrient distribution in response to intake. The metabolic system depends on its signaling. The question is not whether insulin rises, but how exposure is patterned across time.

This pattern exists within a broader timing environment. Sleep cycles, physical activity, muscle mass, circadian alignment, and life stage co-author exposure contour. Insulin does not determine metabolic destiny independently. It functions as one signal among many within an integrated regulatory network.

Long-horizon architecture reframes focus from momentary peaks to repeated contour. It emphasizes continuity over reaction. Adaptation reflects dominant exposure pattern rather than exceptional days.

Insulin exposure, viewed architecturally, is a long-horizon signal pattern shaped by repetition, clearance efficiency, oscillatory integrity, and physiological context—an integrated contour influencing metabolic regulation more through accumulated rhythm than isolated elevation.

Across seasons and life phases, dominant signal environment may shift. Periods of higher activity, altered sleep, or changing hormonal context modify how exposure is processed, yet adaptation still reflects what is most consistent. Months characterized by compressed oscillation create one architectural pattern. Months characterized by clear elevation and descent create another. The body integrates recurring contours rather than storing isolated events.

Receptor responsiveness adjusts gradually in response to repeated exposure. When elevation is frequent and prolonged, receptor dynamics recalibrate to that environment. When oscillation remains distinct and recoverable, responsiveness aligns with that rhythm. These adjustments are incremental, reflecting cumulative experience rather than abrupt transition.

Insulin exposure ultimately functions as a long-horizon regulatory architecture shaped by repeated contour across seasons and life phases, exerting influence through accumulated patterning rather than daily reaction.

Metabolic Flexibility Under Repeated Restriction

Restriction, when applied to feeding timing, functions as a recurring metabolic signal. A single extended interval without intake produces an acute response. When that interval is repeated predictably across days, it becomes a patterned stimulus. The distinction lies not in duration alone, but in recurrence.

Repeated restriction introduces consistent periods during which exogenous energy is unavailable. Over weeks, the metabolic system recalibrates around that expectation. Enzymes supporting substrate mobilization increase in activity during those intervals. Appetite signaling shifts toward the opening of the feeding window. Early energy fluctuations diminish as transitions become more efficient.

Metabolic flexibility can be strengthened through repetition. When the organism repeatedly alternates between intake and the absence of intake, substrate switching becomes less abrupt. The transition from carbohydrate-dominant oxidation to increased reliance on endogenous fuel can occur with reduced perceptual strain. Efficiency gains emerge not from severity, but from rehearsal.

Early exposure often includes disruption. During the first weeks of a new restriction pattern, hunger may appear at previously habitual mealtimes. Energy may feel uneven during fasting intervals. Cognitive focus may fluctuate. As repetition continues and recovery remains sufficient, these disruptions often stabilize. Appetite becomes entrained to the new schedule. Energy oscillations become more predictable. What initially felt abrupt becomes routine.

This stabilization illustrates adaptive recalibration. The system adjusts to what it experiences consistently. Repeated intervals without intake encourage upregulation of pathways supporting substrate mobilization. Glycogen handling becomes more predictable. The transition cost between fed and post-absorptive states may decline.

However, not all outcomes improve simply through repetition. Total energy sufficiency remains a separate variable. If restriction reduces intake below what workload and recovery require, efficiency gains in substrate switching do not offset cumulative deficit. Adaptation to repeated restriction does not eliminate the physiological consequences of sustained underfeeding. The system can become more efficient at mobilizing stored energy without necessarily preserving lean mass or performance under chronic deficit.

The difference between adaptation and escalation becomes relevant here. Adaptation refers to improved efficiency in handling repeated stimuli. Escalation refers to increasing the magnitude or frequency of restriction in pursuit of additional effect. Efficiency gains often plateau once the system recalibrates to the dominant pattern. Extending fasting intervals beyond that point rarely produces proportional improvement. It increases strain.

An example illustrates early disruption followed by stabilization. An individual introduces a consistent daily fasting interval. During the first two weeks, late-morning hunger is pronounced and concentration fluctuates. By the fourth week, hunger shifts toward the scheduled first meal. Morning focus improves as the body anticipates the new pattern. No change in duration occurs; repetition alone alters subjective response. The adaptation reflects improved transition efficiency and appetite entrainment.

An instability pattern can emerge when repetition exceeds recovery capacity. If fasting intervals are layered onto high physical workload without sufficient intake during feeding periods, fatigue may accumulate. Appetite may become exaggerated during meals, or conversely, suppressed despite inadequate intake. Sleep may fragment subtly. The repeated stimulus remains, but recovery between cycles becomes incomplete. Rather than improving flexibility, the system shifts toward conservation.

Chronic low energy availability represents a constraint on adaptation. When total intake remains persistently below expenditure, repeated restriction reinforces deficit. Enzymatic efficiency in mobilizing fuel may increase, yet anabolic processes may downregulate. Reproductive signaling, thyroid activity, or spontaneous movement can adjust downward to conserve energy. These responses are adaptive in a narrow sense, but they reflect conservation rather than expanded flexibility.

Repeated restriction therefore operates within boundaries. When repetition is recoverable—supported by adequate intake, sleep, and workload balance—efficiency in substrate switching and appetite entrainment can improve. When repetition is intensified without regard for sufficiency, adaptation shifts toward protective downregulation.

The metabolic system responds primarily to the pattern most frequently experienced. Repeated restriction, applied consistently and integrated within adequate recovery, can refine transition efficiency. Intensification beyond adaptive range does not guarantee further benefit.

Timing restriction functions as an adaptive stimulus whose effects depend on consistent, recoverable exposure rather than on escalating intensity.

Restriction as a timing signal differs from restriction as an energy deficit. A timing signal reorganizes when intake occurs while preserving sufficient total energy across the cycle. An energy deficit reduces total intake relative to expenditure. The metabolic consequences of these two forms of restriction diverge. Timing-based restriction trains the system to anticipate intervals without intake and to transition efficiently between states. Deficit-based restriction imposes cumulative resource limitation that triggers conservation responses.

Adaptive range refers to the span within which the system can recalibrate without compromising broader function. Within this range, repeated fasting intervals can enhance efficiency in substrate switching and appetite entrainment. Beyond this range, responses shift from optimization to conservation. Energy expenditure may decline modestly. Non-essential processes may be deprioritized. These adjustments are not failures; they are protective recalibrations to sustained scarcity.

Repetition builds efficiency only when oscillation remains intact. Oscillation requires adequate refeeding after each restriction interval. When feeding phases restore glycogen and meet energy demands, the next restriction interval functions as a contained stimulus. When refeeding is incomplete, oscillation narrows. The system begins each cycle from a progressively lower resource state. Over time, flexibility gives way to guarded conservation.

The stimulus–recovery model clarifies this relationship. In exercise physiology, training stimulus produces adaptation only when recovery allows repair and consolidation. Repeated fasting intervals operate similarly. The fasting period acts as stimulus. The feeding period acts as recovery. If recovery is sufficient, transition efficiency improves. If recovery is truncated or energetically inadequate, cumulative strain accumulates.

Metabolic systems also distinguish predictable restriction from unpredictable scarcity. Predictability allows anticipation. Hormonal rhythms align with expected intervals. Appetite cues adjust. Unpredictable scarcity—irregular, variable, or erratic restriction—creates volatility rather than stable adaptation. Consistency reduces uncertainty, which in turn reduces the magnitude of compensatory signaling.

Plateau dynamics often follow consolidation of adaptation. After several weeks of consistent timing, early improvements in transition efficiency and appetite stability may level off. Hunger becomes predictable. Energy fluctuations moderate. Further gains do not necessarily occur with continued repetition of the same pattern. Escalation at this stage does not automatically produce additional efficiency. The system has adapted to the dominant stimulus.

An example illustrates plateau without escalation. An individual adopts a consistent daily fasting interval. Initial weeks bring perceptible changes in hunger rhythm and morning energy stability. By the second month, these changes stabilize. No further improvements in subjective energy are observed despite continued adherence. Extending the fasting interval does not necessarily enhance efficiency; it simply increases stimulus magnitude. The plateau reflects successful adaptation, not stagnation.

Efficiency gains reduce perceptual strain—the sense of abrupt hunger, fatigue, or cognitive disruption during restriction. They do not reduce fundamental caloric needs. Energy requirements remain governed by body size, activity level, and physiological state. Improved tolerance of fasting intervals does not imply reduced need for total intake across the cycle.

Repeated restriction therefore functions within a bounded adaptive framework. When oscillation is preserved and recovery is adequate, efficiency in transition can improve. When recovery capacity or energy sufficiency is compromised, adaptation shifts toward conservation. The stimulus yields benefit only within the limits of recoverable repetition.

Repeated restriction is thus a conditional adaptive stimulus, bounded by recovery capacity and total energy sufficiency, whose benefits emerge from predictable, supported repetition rather than from intensification. That conditionality becomes clearer when the endocrine system is treated as a coordinated network rather than isolated hormones.

Repeated timing restriction does not influence a single hormone in isolation. It interacts with an endocrine network in which signals are interdependent. Insulin, cortisol, thyroid hormones, leptin, and reproductive hormones operate in coordinated rhythm. When feeding timing is altered predictably, this network recalibrates as a system rather than as a collection of independent spikes.

Cortisol follows a diurnal rhythm, typically rising in the early morning and declining toward evening. When fasting intervals are introduced consistently, cortisol may transiently support glucose maintenance during the initial adjustment period. Over repeated cycles, predictability reduces the need for exaggerated compensatory responses. If feeding and fasting intervals remain stable and recovery is adequate, cortisol rhythm often realigns within the new structure. The elevation associated with early adaptation tends to moderate as the body anticipates predictable restriction rather than perceiving it as an acute threat.

Thyroid signaling reflects broader energy availability and recovery sufficiency. Under adequate intake during feeding periods, repeated timing restriction may coexist with stable thyroid output. Metabolic rate remains supported because total energy sufficiency is maintained across the cycle. In contrast, when repeated restriction coincides with chronically low intake, thyroid activity may downshift modestly as part of a conservation response. This modulation is not inherently pathological; it reflects the body's assessment of resource availability over time.

Leptin, produced by adipose tissue, communicates information about energy stores and intake patterns. With consistent timing restriction and adequate caloric repletion, leptin rhythms can stabilize in alignment with feeding windows. Appetite becomes more predictable. When restriction is layered onto insufficient intake, leptin levels may decline persistently, intensifying hunger signals and narrowing hormonal range. The distinction lies in whether repetition occurs within sufficient energy support.

Reproductive signaling is particularly sensitive to sustained low energy availability. In individuals with adequate intake and recovery, repeated timing restriction may integrate without significant disruption to reproductive hormones. However, when energy availability falls below individual thresholds, reproductive signaling may adjust downward as a protective measure. This sensitivity can be more pronounced in females, whose hormonal milieu responds closely to energy sufficiency. The modulation reflects systemic prioritization rather than isolated dysfunction.

An example of stable integration illustrates coordinated hormonal adjustment. An individual introduces a consistent fasting interval while maintaining total caloric adequacy and stable sleep. Initial fluctuations in hunger and morning alertness settle over several weeks. Cortisol rhythm aligns with the new feeding pattern. Thyroid output remains stable. Leptin fluctuations become predictable around meals. The endocrine network adapts collectively, not through exaggerated spikes but through coordinated recalibration.

An instability pattern emerges when repeated restriction is combined with inadequate recovery. If caloric intake remains insufficient and sleep becomes inconsistent, thyroid signaling may trend downward, leptin may decline, and reproductive hormones may become less stable. Cortisol rhythm may lose its diurnal clarity. These changes reflect protective downregulation rather than adaptive modulation. The system is responding to cumulative resource strain, not to timing alone.

Predictability plays a central role in hormonal integration. When feeding and fasting intervals are consistent, endocrine responses become anticipatory rather than reactive. Appetite cues align. Cortisol peaks become rhythmic rather than erratic. The network operates within a narrower, more stable range. Unpredictable or excessively intensified restriction, by contrast, increases variability across the network.

The distinction between adaptive modulation and protective downregulation clarifies interpretation. Adaptive modulation refers to subtle recalibration within functional range—more efficient substrate switching, stabilized appetite rhythm, preserved thyroid activity under adequate intake. Protective downregulation reflects conservation in response to sustained insufficiency—reduced metabolic output, suppressed reproductive signaling, amplified hunger.

Repeated timing restriction therefore interacts with endocrine systems in a context-dependent manner. Hormonal responses reflect the combined influence of timing predictability, total energy availability, sleep integrity, and individual sensitivity. No single hormone dictates the outcome; the network adapts collectively to the dominant pattern.

Hormonal integration under repeated timing restriction is best understood as context-dependent modulation within a coordinated endocrine system rather than as automatic harm or guaranteed optimization.

Hormones function as networked regulators of resource allocation. Insulin signals nutrient availability. Cortisol supports mobilization when intake is absent or demand rises. Thyroid hormones influence metabolic rate and cellular energy throughput. Reproductive hormones respond to perceived resource sufficiency. These axes communicate through feedback loops rather than operating independently. A shift in one domain influences others through shared regulatory pathways.

For example, sustained low leptin signaling—reflecting reduced energy availability—can influence thyroid conversion and reproductive signaling. Cortisol patterns may adjust in response to changes in sleep or energy status, indirectly modifying glucose handling and appetite. Insulin exposure interacts with these systems by shaping substrate availability across time. The organism interprets cumulative signals, not isolated elevations.

Predictable timing reduces neuroendocrine uncertainty. When feeding and fasting intervals are consistent and total intake remains sufficient, the endocrine network can anticipate energy flux. Cortisol peaks align with expected fasting phases. Appetite hormones cluster around feeding windows. Thyroid output remains proportionate to overall energy status.

Stability emerges not because restriction is absent, but because the pattern is coherent and supported.

Acute stress responses differ structurally from chronic conservation. In early exposure to timing restriction, transient increases in mobilizing hormones may occur as the body adjusts to new intervals. When recovery is adequate, these responses moderate as predictability increases. Chronic conservation, by contrast, reflects cumulative insufficiency. Thyroid signaling may trend downward gradually. Reproductive hormones may become less robust. These changes develop over months, not days, and reflect persistent resource limitation rather than the mere presence of fasting intervals.

Hormonal range narrowing is typically incremental. The system does not abruptly collapse into dysfunction when restriction begins. Instead, subtle shifts accumulate if energy sufficiency is not restored consistently. Slight reductions in metabolic rate, mild changes in cycle regularity, or increased hunger intensity may appear gradually. These represent integrated network responses to sustained deficit.

Body fat level also influences endocrine response to restriction. Higher fat mass often corresponds with higher baseline leptin, which may buffer short-term restriction without immediate hormonal downregulation. Lower body fat reduces this buffer. In leaner individuals, repeated restriction combined with insufficient intake may more readily influence reproductive and thyroid signaling. The timing pattern itself remains constant; available energy reserves alter system interpretation.

An example of hormonal stability under adequate recovery involves an individual maintaining consistent feeding timing while ensuring sufficient caloric intake and stable sleep. Over months, appetite rhythm stabilizes. Thyroid output remains within normal range. Menstrual cycles remain regular. Cortisol retains diurnal clarity. The network has integrated timing without narrowing range.

By contrast, subtle downregulation may unfold when repeated restriction coincides with chronic underfeeding. Over several months, resting energy expenditure may decrease slightly. Cycle length may vary. Hunger cues may intensify despite adherence to timing. These changes reflect cumulative deficit. The destabilizing variable is not timing alone, but sustained resource shortfall.

Timing serves as a patterning input. Endocrine response reflects the integrated signal of timing plus total energy availability, sleep, and body composition. When recovery and intake are proportionate, hormonal modulation remains within adaptive range. When cumulative deficit dominates, protective adjustments gradually narrow that range.

Endocrine response to repeated timing restriction is therefore pattern-sensitive and recovery-dependent, shaped by the combined influence of energy sufficiency, sleep integrity, body composition, and consistent exposure rather than by fasting intervals alone.

Timing restriction does not occur in isolation from the rest of life. It intersects with physical workload, cognitive demand, psychological stress, and sleep quality. These factors collectively define total load. Adaptive capacity can be understood as finite bandwidth—the amount of strain the system can absorb while maintaining coherence.

When timing restriction is introduced into a context of moderate load and adequate recovery, integration is often stable. Physical activity is proportionate. Cognitive demands fluctuate within a manageable range. Sleep remains consistent. Under these conditions, the organism can allocate sufficient resources to both daily function and adaptation to repeated restriction. Oscillation remains intact. Recovery between cycles is adequate.

However, load stacking alters this equation. Load stacking occurs when multiple stressors converge: increased training volume, occupational pressure, reduced sleep, and repeated fasting intervals layered simultaneously. Each factor independently demands adaptive resources. Together, they compress recovery margin.

Recovery margin refers to the difference between total load and total capacity. When margin is wide, variability is tolerated. When margin narrows, the system becomes less resilient to additional strain. Timing restriction that was previously integrated without difficulty may begin to feel destabilizing under stacked load.

For example, an individual practicing consistent timing restriction while engaging in moderate resistance training and maintaining stable sleep may experience steady energy and appetite rhythm. If training volume increases substantially—such as adding endurance sessions or preparing for competition—without a corresponding change in feeding structure or sleep duration, recovery demand rises. The same fasting interval now occurs in a higher-load environment. Energy fluctuations may become more pronounced. Perceived exertion may increase. Appetite volatility may intensify.

An instability pattern emerges when load stacking persists. Training stress combined with cognitive pressure and reduced sleep can gradually narrow adaptive window. Early signs may be subtle: delayed recovery between sessions, increased irritability during fasting intervals, greater hunger intensity late in the feeding window, or mild sleep fragmentation. None of these signs indicate immediate failure. They signal compression of bandwidth.

Sleep compression acts as a particularly significant recovery constraint. Reduced sleep impairs physical recovery, cognitive performance, and metabolic regulation. When sleep duration declines, the system has fewer hours for restoration. Timing restriction layered onto compressed sleep reduces opportunity for full recalibration between cycles. Even if total caloric intake remains stable, reduced recovery time alters tolerance.

High training volume introduces another constraint. Endurance athletes or individuals engaged in heavy manual labor expend substantial energy daily. Muscle repair and glycogen replenishment require adequate intake and rest. When fasting intervals reduce the window available for replenishment and total intake does not fully compensate, recovery may lag. The timing pattern itself remains unchanged; the environment in which it operates has shifted.

The difference between tolerable and destabilizing restriction lies in available bandwidth. Under moderate load, restriction coexists with stable performance. Under stacked load and compressed recovery, identical restriction narrows flexibility. The structure remains constant; capacity does not.

Cumulative strain often develops gradually. Weeks of stacked load may pass before noticeable shifts appear. Energy may decline incrementally. Motivation for training may waver. Hunger patterns may become less predictable. These changes reflect adaptive window narrowing rather than abrupt breakdown.

Importantly, timing restriction does not inherently create instability under load. It interacts with the sum of demands. In some contexts, a defined feeding window may simplify scheduling under high workload by consolidating decisions. In others, it may reduce available margin when recovery is already limited.

Adaptive capacity is dynamic. It expands during periods of balanced load and contracts when strain accumulates. Recognizing that restriction consumes part of this capacity clarifies why identical timing patterns behave differently across contexts. The organism integrates total load, not isolated variables.

When total load approaches or exceeds capacity, restriction becomes one variable too many.

Repeated timing restriction is therefore sustainable only within available recovery bandwidth and total load tolerance, functioning effectively when integrated into—rather than layered onto—the broader demands of life.

Adaptive bandwidth is not fixed. It expands and contracts in response to training status, sleep quality, psychological environment, and seasonal demands. Periods of balanced workload and sufficient recovery often widen this bandwidth, allowing greater tolerance for structured restriction. Periods of intensified demand narrow it. The same fasting interval may feel neutral in one phase and destabilizing in another because capacity has shifted.

Metabolic load and neural load interact continuously. Physical training imposes metabolic demand through substrate turnover and tissue repair. Cognitive and psychological stress impose neural demand through sustained sympathetic activation and attentional strain. Although these forms of load differ in origin, they draw from overlapping recovery resources—sleep, caloric sufficiency, and autonomic balance. When neural load increases substantially, tolerance for additional metabolic challenge may decline even if physical workload remains unchanged.

Energy flux and recovery time represent distinct dimensions. High energy flux—substantial intake matched by substantial expenditure—can coexist with robust adaptation when recovery time is adequate. Conversely, moderate energy flux paired with insufficient sleep or constant cognitive demand can narrow recovery margin. Timing restriction interacts with both dimensions. It modifies when intake occurs, but its impact depends on whether energy flux and recovery time remain proportionate.

Micro-strain accumulation often unfolds quietly. Each day of slightly reduced recovery or marginally elevated demand may not produce noticeable change. Over weeks, however, small discrepancies accumulate. Morning alertness may decline subtly. Training performance may plateau earlier in sessions. Appetite patterns may become less predictable. These shifts are gradual and easily attributed to routine variability. Yet they signal erosion of adaptive window rather than isolated fatigue.

Fatigue and adaptive window narrowing are related but not identical. Fatigue reflects acute or short-term depletion that resolves with rest. Adaptive window narrowing reflects reduced tolerance for variation—less capacity to absorb additional load without destabilization. An individual may feel only mildly fatigued yet exhibit increased sensitivity to fasting intervals or meal timing shifts. The system's buffer has contracted even if overt exhaustion is absent.

Metabolic systems triage resources under stacked demand. When energy and recovery are limited relative to load, priority is given to essential functions: maintaining blood glucose, supporting vital organs, and preserving immediate survival capacity. Secondary processes—optimal performance output, robust reproductive signaling, or maximal metabolic rate—may be downregulated temporarily. Timing restriction introduced into this environment competes for limited adaptive resources.

Consider an individual during a moderate training phase: three weekly resistance sessions, stable sleep, manageable work stress. Timing restriction integrates smoothly. Transition efficiency is maintained. Appetite rhythm is predictable. During a peak training phase—higher volume, added conditioning, travel demands—the same timing pattern may begin to feel more taxing. Recovery between sessions lags. Hunger intensity increases late in the window. No change in fasting duration has occurred; total load has increased.

Similarly, an individual with stable physical load but escalating cognitive workload—extended deadlines, prolonged concentration, emotional stress—may find that previously tolerable fasting intervals now produce irritability or diminished focus. Physical expenditure remains constant. Neural demand has increased. Recovery margin contracts despite unchanged training.

In each case, timing restriction becomes destabilizing only when it competes with insufficient recovery. The fasting interval itself has not changed. The context into which it is placed has shifted.

Adaptive limits therefore depend on the balance between total load and available recovery. When bandwidth is sufficient, repeated restriction can integrate without strain. When bandwidth narrows, identical restriction can exceed tolerance. The constraint is not inherent to the fasting interval but to the load-sensitive capacity of the system.

Adaptive limits are thus load-dependent and context-sensitive, shaped by the dynamic interplay of metabolic, neural, and recovery demands rather than by fasting duration alone.

Repeated timing restriction is not only a metabolic pattern. It is a cognitive pattern. Over time, the structure is interpreted, narrated internally, and integrated into self-concept. These psychological processes alter total load without altering caloric intake.

Perception functions as a regulatory variable. Hunger, for example, is a physiological signal indicating the absence of recent intake. The sensation itself is not inherently destabilizing. It becomes destabilizing or neutral depending on interpretation. When hunger is processed as an expected phase within a structured interval, sympathetic activation may remain modest. The signal is informational. When interpreted as deprivation or loss of control, the same sensation may elevate arousal. Cortical evaluation modifies autonomic tone. The caloric pattern is unchanged; the internal response differs.

Structure can operate as a stabilizing scaffold. Defined feeding boundaries reduce moment-to-moment decision-making. Cognitive bandwidth is preserved because fewer choices require evaluation. Appetite signals align predictably with anticipated intake. This alignment reduces uncertainty.

The same structure can shift toward internal surveillance. When attention narrows excessively toward compliance, minor deviations acquire disproportionate meaning. A delayed meal—even by minutes—may generate elevated internal monitoring. Intake remains the same. Psychological load increases. Surveillance consumes bandwidth.

Repeated exposure often moves behavior toward identity integration. What begins as "a pattern I follow" becomes "how I eat." Identity consolidation reduces decision fatigue. Fewer deliberations are required because the behavior is no longer negotiated. Stability increases. Appetite entrainment aligns more smoothly with expectation. The pattern feels automatic rather than effortful.

This consolidation supports adherence under moderate load. It can also reduce flexibility when overextended. When timing becomes part of self-description, deviation may be experienced as a threat to coherence. The behavior is no longer simply structural; it is symbolic. Contextual variability then requires not only behavioral adjustment but identity adjustment.

Consider an individual who has practiced consistent timing restriction for a year. During a period of increased occupational workload, daily schedule shifts unpredictably. If identity remains flexible, the individual adjusts meal timing within broader boundaries without distress and returns to baseline structure when workload normalizes. The pattern is preserved, but flexibility absorbs variability. Psychological load remains stable.

Contrast this with an individual whose timing structure is tightly bound to identity. Under similar workload changes, small deviations provoke disproportionate discomfort. Internal narrative frames disruption as regression. Intake and metabolic contour remain similar. Distress rises because rigidity amplifies interpretation.

Escalation drift often emerges after adaptation plateau. Initial weeks of repeated restriction produce noticeable changes—hunger predictability, energy stability. Over months, adaptation consolidates. Subjective novelty diminishes. Plateau appears. Plateau is often interpreted as insufficiency rather than completion of adaptation.

From this interpretation, incremental extension follows. The feeding window narrows slightly. Adaptation restabilizes. Later, further narrowing occurs. Each change appears modest. Because prior adaptation reduced perceptual strain, further intensification feels manageable. Recovery margin compresses quietly.

Across several months, escalation drift can unfold without overt instability. An individual may reduce a ten-hour window to eight, then to six. No dramatic symptoms appear. However, subtle shifts accumulate: increased preoccupation with timing precision, sharper hunger intensity near the window boundary, slightly reduced tolerance for workload variation. Each intensification consumes bandwidth incrementally.

Escalation does not guarantee improved efficiency. Once oscillatory adaptation consolidates, further compression increases intensity, not flexibility. The system has already learned the pattern; additional restriction narrows margin without enhancing regulation.

Two self-reinforcing loops illustrate divergent trajectories.

Stable Integration Loop:

Predictable timing → reduced decision fatigue → stable appetite rhythm → flexible identity → maintained recovery margin → sustained repetition without intensification.

This loop stabilizes without requiring escalation. Plateau is interpreted as equilibrium rather than insufficiency.

Escalation Drift Loop:

Adaptation plateau → interpretation as stagnation → incremental restriction → slight bandwidth compression → subtle strain → interpretation of strain as insufficient discipline → further restriction.

The loop tightens gradually.

Rigidity further amplifies psychological load even when metabolic contour remains stable. An individual may maintain identical intake and timing yet experience rising distress due to hyper-focus on adherence. The pattern itself is not destabilizing. The internal surveillance surrounding it increases sympathetic tone and reduces cognitive flexibility.

A six-hour window experienced as structured flexibility differs from the same window experienced as a non-negotiable identity marker. The metabolic input is identical. The perceptual overlay modifies total load.

Repeated timing restriction is structurally neutral architecture. Its long-term stability depends less on duration than on perceptual framing, identity flexibility, and the absence of gradual escalation drift.

Perception does not merely color experience; it alters load distribution. When a structured fasting interval is framed as chosen and bounded, sympathetic activation tends to remain proportionate. The organism anticipates the interval as finite. When the same interval is framed as compulsory or fragile, anticipatory vigilance increases. Vigilance consumes bandwidth. Even if caloric intake and timing remain identical, internal monitoring of adherence increases cognitive strain. Over weeks, this additional load can narrow tolerance for variation without any measurable metabolic shift.

Identity consolidation similarly alters recovery dynamics. When behavior integrates into identity, compliance requires less conscious effort. This reduces acute decision fatigue. However, identity-bound behaviors resist contextual modification because deviation carries symbolic weight. A flexible identity absorbs variation by distinguishing structure from self-worth. A rigid identity conflates structure with coherence. In the latter case, minor timing disruptions trigger disproportionate cognitive processing. Energy expenditure rises not through metabolic demand, but through evaluative load.

Escalation drift compresses margin gradually because adaptation masks intensity. As perceptual strain declines with repetition, additional compression feels neutral at first. The system has already recalibrated to oscillation. When the feeding window narrows further, the immediate subjective response may be minimal. Yet each incremental compression reduces temporal flexibility. Fewer hours remain available for repletion. Fewer scheduling deviations can be absorbed without friction. The narrowing occurs at the level of optionality before it appears at the level of overt fatigue.

Over time, the distinction between voluntary refinement and compulsive tightening can blur internally. Because each adjustment is modest, escalation can be interpreted as optimization. Recovery margin erodes in small increments. Flexibility declines before dysfunction appears. This is why escalation drift is often detected not by dramatic symptoms, but by reduced tolerance for disruption.

The divergence between stable integration and the escalation loop is therefore not defined by duration alone, but by interpretive framing. In stable integration, plateau signals consolidation. In escalation drift, plateau signals insufficiency. The physiological pattern may be identical at the outset. The trajectory diverges through interpretation.

Psychological rigidity increases total load even when caloric structure remains constant because vigilance amplifies sympathetic tone. Elevated monitoring reduces cognitive flexibility and increases reactivity to minor deviation. This additional load can interact with physical or occupational stress, narrowing bandwidth further without any change in fasting duration.

Timing architecture therefore exerts its long-term influence through interaction with perception and identity. When framing remains neutral and identity remains flexible, repetition stabilizes. When escalation drift narrows margin and rigidity increases monitoring load, stability erodes gradually.

Repeated timing restriction remains viable architecture when perceptual load is proportionate, identity is flexible, and escalation does not compress recovery bandwidth beyond contextual tolerance.

Over extended periods, repeated timing restriction can shift from active adaptation to structural consolidation. Consolidation does not imply intensification. It reflects stabilization of pattern without further tightening. The feeding structure becomes predictable, oscillation remains intact, and recovery remains proportionate. The pattern persists without requiring progressive compression.

Consolidation is often misinterpreted as stagnation. In structural terms, it represents equilibrium. The system has adapted to the dominant exposure contour. Appetite rhythm aligns with timing. Energy transitions feel familiar rather than disruptive. No additional efficiency is gained through further restriction, yet no additional strain is imposed. Stability replaces novelty.

Long-horizon stability depends less on daily precision and more on pattern density across weeks and seasons. Pattern density refers to how consistently a given structure is repeated relative to deviations. A structure repeated most days across months defines the dominant architectural signal. Occasional deviations—extended meals during travel, altered timing during holidays, schedule shifts during seasonal workload changes—rarely dismantle this architecture.

Temporal elasticity within stable boundaries supports resilience. Elasticity refers to the capacity to absorb short-term variability without destabilizing long-term pattern. When oscillation remains recoverable and total intake remains proportionate, occasional expansion or compression of a feeding window does not erase adaptation. The system responds primarily to repeated contour, not isolated days.

For example, an individual maintains a consistent daily feeding window across most of the year. During summer months, physical activity increases and social events shift meal timing slightly later. The window occasionally expands by one to two hours. With the return to regular schedule in autumn, original timing resumes without difficulty. Appetite rhythm realigns quickly. No structural reset is required. The dominant multi-year pattern remains intact.

Similarly, a single day of early-morning intake during travel does not dismantle adaptation developed over months. Oscillation resumes once regular timing returns. Architecture reflects cumulative repetition, not episodic deviation.

Structural continuity differs from numerical precision. Continuity refers to maintaining a coherent rhythm across time. Precision refers to exact minute-by-minute adherence. Long-term stability depends more on continuity than on precision. Minor fluctuations in start or end times do not materially alter exposure architecture when the broader pattern remains consistent.

Contrast this with an escalated pattern characterized by progressive tightening. In such a pattern, stability depends on maintaining increasingly narrow parameters. Variability tolerance decreases. A single deviation feels disruptive because recovery margin is limited. Consolidated patterns tolerate variability without destabilization; escalated patterns require strict maintenance to avoid strain.

Seasonal variability often reveals the robustness of consolidation. During periods of lower workload, appetite may shift slightly earlier or later without difficulty. During periods of higher workload, meal distribution within the window may adjust modestly. If recovery remains adequate, the core structure absorbs these fluctuations. Stability is preserved because oscillation across months remains coherent.

Receptor responsiveness, enzymatic activity, and appetite entrainment respond to the dominant pattern. A brief interruption does not override months of patterned exposure. Only sustained alteration of contour reshapes adaptation.

Consolidation therefore represents the point at which timing restriction functions as background structure rather than active stimulus. The pattern persists without intensification. Variability tolerance signals resilience. Recovery alignment across months maintains oscillatory integrity.

Repeated timing restriction becomes durable when consolidation preserves flexibility, variability is absorbed without strain, and oscillation remains recoverable across seasons. Long-horizon stability depends on proportional alignment and tolerance for deviation rather than on numerical rigidity within isolated days.

Long-horizon stability also depends on oscillatory integrity across shifting life phases. Consolidation does not imply static repetition under identical conditions. Workload changes, aging, training phases, travel, and seasonal daylight variation alter the surrounding environment in which timing operates. A consolidated structure demonstrates resilience by remaining recognizable across these shifts without requiring escalation. The feeding window may flex modestly, meal density may adjust, but the underlying rhythm persists.

Durability emerges from recoverable oscillation, not from maximal compression. When feeding and fasting phases continue to alternate with adequate restoration, the architecture remains intact. If variability is absorbed without disproportionate strain, flexibility is preserved. This preservation reflects sufficient recovery margin rather than strict precision.

Consolidation also alters psychological demand. Once structure becomes background, monitoring decreases. Timing requires less vigilance. The absence of continual negotiation reduces sympathetic activation associated with adherence. The pattern exists without constant evaluation. This reduction in evaluative load distinguishes durable consolidation from rigid maintenance.

In contrast, escalated patterns often rely on sustained vigilance. As windows narrow progressively, tolerance for deviation declines. The structure requires active enforcement rather than passive integration. Over time, this enforcement increases total load even if caloric intake remains adequate. Stability becomes conditional on maintaining increasingly narrow parameters. Variability tolerance diminishes.

A pattern repeated consistently across years, even with seasonal variation, exerts stronger regulatory influence than intermittent periods of intense restriction followed by disruption. Density of repetition outweighs severity of compression.

Variability tolerance therefore functions as a resilience marker. A consolidated structure can expand slightly during social periods and contract modestly during focused phases without destabilization. The system recognizes the broader contour as continuous. Oscillation resumes predictably because the dominant rhythm has been reinforced repeatedly.

Only sustained alteration of contour reshapes architecture. A brief period of extended intake does not dismantle months of structured timing. Likewise, a short interval of intensified restriction does not permanently enhance efficiency if the dominant pattern remains unchanged. Adaptation reflects what is most frequent, not what is most extreme.

Consolidation preserves recovery bandwidth, maintains variability tolerance, and keeps oscillation recoverable across seasons and life phases.

Durability arises from proportion and pattern density rather than from maximal compression within isolated days.

Hormonal Signaling and Stress Load

Energy availability is not simply a calorie total. It is a systemic signal reflecting the proportion between intake and expenditure across time. The organism interprets this proportion as information about environmental sufficiency. Timing restriction modifies when energy enters the system. Energy availability determines whether sufficient energy enters at all.

The distinction between timing restriction and energy deficit is structural. Timing restriction reorganizes intake across hours. Energy deficit reflects a sustained mismatch between total intake and total expenditure. These variables often overlap but are not equivalent. A compressed feeding window can coexist with adequate energy availability. Conversely, frequent meals can still result in deficit if intake remains insufficient.

Energy availability operates as proportion rather than as a raw number. A given caloric intake may be adequate during a sedentary phase and inadequate during high training volume. Expenditure varies with physical activity, occupational demand, and spontaneous movement. Resource signaling reflects this dynamic relationship rather than intake alone.

Across repeated cycles, the balance between mobilization and restoration determines long-term stability. Mobilization draws from stored substrates during fasting intervals or periods of energy demand. Restoration replenishes those stores during feeding. When mobilization and restoration remain proportionate, oscillation supports flexibility without eroding reserves. When mobilization consistently exceeds restoration, deficit accumulates quietly.

Short-term tolerance can obscure long-term insufficiency. The body can compensate for modest deficit over days or weeks without overt disruption. Appetite may recalibrate. Energy output may adjust subtly. Perceived adaptation—greater comfort during fasting intervals, reduced hunger intensity—can coexist with gradual resource erosion if intake does not match expenditure.

Efficiency does not eliminate requirement. Improved substrate switching may make fasting intervals feel smoother. Appetite entrainment may reduce perceived strain. These adaptations reflect improved handling of timing restriction, not reduced energy needs. Tissue repair, immune function, reproductive signaling, and cognitive performance continue to require adequate substrate.

Consider an individual practicing consistent timing restriction while maintaining sufficient caloric intake relative to moderate physical workload. Meals within the window restore glycogen and meet energy demand. Body weight remains stable. Training performance is preserved. Appetite rhythm aligns with schedule. Energy availability remains proportionate, allowing timing restriction to function as structural organization rather than deficit.

Contrast this with an individual layering repeated timing restriction onto marginal intake during increased training volume. Meals within the window do not fully replenish glycogen. Recovery between sessions lengthens. Resting energy expenditure may decline subtly. Hunger cues may oscillate unpredictably. The feeding window remains intact, but resource signaling reflects insufficiency. The adaptation observed—tolerance of fasting intervals—masks a narrowing margin.

Apparent stability can therefore conceal slow deficit. Body weight may change minimally in early phases due to compensatory reductions in spontaneous movement or metabolic rate. Energy may feel adequate during routine tasks while performance capacity declines gradually. Because timing structure remains consistent, instability may be attributed elsewhere. Yet the underlying variable is cumulative under-restoration.

Resource signaling integrates across weeks. Leptin trends, thyroid modulation, and reproductive signaling reflect sustained proportion rather than isolated days. The organism evaluates dominant patterns. If restoration routinely meets demand, flexibility is preserved. If restoration lags consistently, conservation responses emerge incrementally.

Metabolic flexibility differs from chronic scarcity. Flexibility involves efficient transition between states with preserved capacity for restoration. Scarcity reflects repeated mobilization without sufficient repletion. Both may produce tolerance to fasting intervals, but their long-term trajectories diverge.

Repeated timing restriction interacts with energy availability as a governing constraint. When intake proportionately matches expenditure across cycles, restriction can refine rhythmic organization. When intake persistently falls short, the same restriction pattern contributes to narrowing capacity over time.

Energy availability ultimately determines whether timing restriction enhances regulatory flexibility or gradually erodes systemic margin. It governs whether mobilization and restoration remain balanced across repeated cycles, shaping long-term capacity more decisively than timing structure alone.

Energy availability functions as background architecture rather than foreground sensation. The organism does not respond to single-day arithmetic. It responds to repeated proportion. A brief mismatch between intake and expenditure can be absorbed without structural change. Sustained mismatch recalibrates allocation priorities. This recalibration often occurs without acute alarm.

Allocation under adequate availability supports both immediate demand and long-term maintenance. Tissue repair, connective integrity, immune surveillance, reproductive signaling, and cognitive resilience operate concurrently with daily output. When availability remains proportionate, these systems proceed without needing to compete aggressively for resources. Oscillation between mobilization and restoration remains balanced.

When availability narrows persistently, resource triage begins gradually. Immediate survival and essential metabolic stability are preserved. Secondary processes may downshift subtly. Recovery between training sessions lengthens slightly. Sleep depth may decline modestly. Motivation for spontaneous movement may decrease. These shifts are not abrupt failures. They reflect incremental conservation in response to sustained proportion mismatch.

The distinction between flexibility and scarcity becomes clearer over longer horizons. In flexible systems, mobilization during fasting is followed by reliable restoration during feeding. Glycogen replenishment occurs predictably. Training output remains stable across weeks. Appetite rhythm aligns with workload. In scarcity, mobilization continues to function, but restoration remains incomplete. Each cycle begins from a slightly reduced reserve state. The reduction may be small enough to avoid immediate detection, yet large enough to accumulate across months.

Efficiency in substrate switching can obscure this process. Improved comfort during fasting does not imply sufficient restoration afterward. An individual may report stable energy during morning fasting intervals while simultaneously experiencing gradual decline in training intensity or cognitive sharpness later in the day. Perceived smoothness of fasting is not equivalent to systemic sufficiency.

Energy availability also interacts with variability tolerance. When reserves are proportionate, occasional expansion of the feeding window or temporary increases in activity can be absorbed without disruption. When reserves are marginal, even minor deviations amplify strain. Tolerance for fluctuation narrows. What was previously absorbed becomes destabilizing.

The governing constraint therefore lies not in the compression of timing, but in the balance of mobilization and restoration across repeated cycles. Timing restriction reorganizes when energy enters the system. Energy availability determines whether enough energy enters to sustain full-spectrum function.

Repeated timing restriction enhances regulatory rhythm only when restoration remains adequate across cycles. When restoration consistently lags behind mobilization, restriction becomes one variable within a broader scarcity signal. Over time, capacity narrows not because of the fasting interval itself, but because cumulative proportion has shifted.

Energy within the human organism is not distributed evenly across systems. It is allocated according to hierarchy. At the base of this hierarchy are processes essential for immediate survival—maintenance of cellular gradients, cardiac rhythm, respiration, and neurological integrity. Above this tier are functions supporting movement, cognition, and environmental interaction. Higher still are reproduction, growth, and long-term repair. At the outer edge are optional enhancements—peak athletic output, maximal muscle accretion, and surplus reproductive robustness.

When energy availability is proportionate to expenditure across time, allocation flows smoothly across tiers. Essential processes are maintained, performance is supported, repair proceeds, and reproductive signaling remains stable. Surplus energy can be directed toward adaptation and resilience. Timing restriction layered onto adequate availability does not disrupt this hierarchy because restoration consistently meets mobilization.

When restoration repeatedly lags behind mobilization, allocation priorities shift. The organism does not abruptly fail. It reallocates.

Hierarchical prioritization under marginal availability is adaptive. Essential survival processes remain protected. Performance and optional processes become negotiable. Long-term repair may slow. Reproductive signaling may attenuate. These changes are not pathological in origin; they reflect intelligent resource management under perceived scarcity.

The shift from optimization to conservation is gradual. Optimization directs available energy toward growth, repair, and performance beyond baseline requirements. Conservation redirects energy toward essential maintenance while trimming discretionary output. The transition is often subtle and unfolds across weeks or months.

Micro-adjustments in resting expenditure illustrate this shift. Under sustained mismatch between intake and expenditure, resting metabolic rate may decline modestly. The change is rarely dramatic enough to be noticed day to day. It accumulates over time as a small percentage adjustment. Spontaneous physical activity—fidgeting, posture changes, incidental movement—may decrease unconsciously. These shifts reduce total expenditure without overt fatigue.

Conservation can occur without acute exhaustion. An individual may feel generally functional while experiencing slight reductions in maximal output. Training sessions may feel marginally more demanding. Recovery between sessions may lengthen. These changes reflect reprioritization rather than collapse.

Performance decline often precedes weight change. Because body mass is influenced by multiple compartments—water, glycogen, lean tissue, fat—short-term stability does not confirm resource sufficiency. The organism may reduce performance output before reducing mass. It preserves structural tissue while trimming discretionary energy use.

Consider an example of adequate allocation. An individual practices timing restriction while maintaining proportionate intake relative to moderate training volume. Glycogen stores are replenished within feeding windows. Sleep remains stable. Performance metrics hold steady across months. Recovery markers remain consistent. Energy allocation flows across tiers without restriction. Conservation responses are unnecessary.

Contrast this with repeated marginal intake layered onto high physical demand. Feeding windows restore some but not all expended energy. Over months, maximal training output declines slightly. Resting energy expenditure decreases modestly. Appetite may fluctuate unpredictably. Body weight remains stable due to compensatory reductions in spontaneous movement. The organism has shifted toward conservation without overt dysfunction.

An illustration clarifies the distinction between acute fatigue and allocation reprioritization. Acute fatigue arises after an unusually demanding session or brief sleep disruption. It resolves with recovery. Allocation reprioritization persists even after short rest because it reflects cumulative pattern. Training output may plateau despite adequate sleep on a given night because the broader energy proportion across weeks remains marginal.

Short-term energy smoothing—feeling steady during fasting intervals—does not guarantee long-term allocation sufficiency. The body can maintain stable glucose and perceived energy through efficient mobilization even while gradually reducing discretionary outputs. Smoothing reflects improved handling of timing. Allocation shift reflects systemic response to proportion.

Gradual narrowing of optional processes often precedes overt metabolic signals. Reproductive robustness may attenuate subtly. Immune resilience may fluctuate. Recovery from minor illness may lengthen. None of these changes necessarily present as dramatic events. They reflect tiered prioritization.

Importantly, conservation responses are adaptive rather than inherently negative. They preserve core function during scarcity. The concern is not the presence of conservation but the context in which it persists. If marginal availability becomes the dominant pattern, reprioritization stabilizes at a lower output level.

Body weight stability does not negate this shift. Stable mass can coexist with reduced performance, slower recovery, and narrowed discretionary energy allocation. The hierarchy is dynamic. It responds to sustained proportion between intake and expenditure.

Timing restriction interacts with this hierarchy indirectly. When restoration within feeding windows matches mobilization demands, allocation remains balanced. When restoration consistently lags—even slightly—hierarchical reprioritization emerges gradually.

Energy allocation hierarchy therefore acts as the mechanism through which sustained availability proportion determines long-term trajectory. Adequate proportion preserves flexibility and full-tier output. Marginal proportion narrows optional processes while protecting essential survival.

Energy allocation is not an all-or-nothing switch. It is a layered prioritization system responding to dominant patterns of availability. Whether timing restriction enhances flexibility or contributes to gradual capacity reprioritization depends on how consistently restoration meets mobilization across repeated cycles.

Performance capacity represents one of the earliest variables to narrow when resource availability trends marginal across time. Unlike essential maintenance processes, performance exists within a discretionary tier. The organism can reduce output without compromising immediate survival. For this reason, performance decline often precedes overt structural breakdown.

Performance capacity differs from baseline functioning. Baseline functioning refers to the ability to conduct daily activities, maintain stable mood, and complete routine tasks. Capacity refers to the ceiling of output—maximal strength, sustained endurance, cognitive throughput under high demand, and adaptive response to training stimulus. When allocation reprioritizes subtly, the ceiling lowers before the floor collapses.

An individual may feel stable in daily life while maximal output drifts downward. Energy may feel even across fasting intervals. Appetite may remain predictable. Body weight may appear unchanged. Yet peak performance metrics—lifting numbers, interval pace, cognitive endurance—may plateau or regress gradually.

This divergence reflects hidden conservation.

Under proportionate intake relative to demand, performance capacity is preserved. Training stimulus generates adaptation. Recovery kinetics remain efficient. Cognitive performance sustains intensity across prolonged tasks. Minor fatigue resolves predictably. In this environment, timing restriction can coexist with robust output because restoration matches mobilization across cycles.

Contrast this with subtle mismatch layered across weeks. Intake remains slightly below cumulative demand. Day-level compensation masks the discrepancy. On any single day, glycogen restoration appears adequate. Subjective energy feels acceptable. However, week-level drift begins to appear. Training output declines marginally from prior baselines. Recovery between sessions lengthens in small increments. Performance variability increases.

This drift rarely appears abrupt. Instead, maximal lifts plateau unexpectedly. Endurance pace requires greater effort. Adaptation to training stimulus slows. These changes are often attributed to programming, sleep variability, or random fluctuation. Yet sustained marginal availability reduces discretionary allocation toward performance adaptation.

Cognitive performance follows similar patterns. Under mild but persistent resource constraint, the ability to sustain deep concentration over extended periods narrows. Daily functioning remains intact. Tasks are completed. However, complex problem-solving capacity or prolonged focus declines subtly. The individual can function but struggles to progress at prior intensity.

Temporal modeling clarifies this progression.

Day-level compensation:

Short-term deficit can be absorbed through increased mobilization of stored substrates. Energy feels stable. Performance appears unaffected.

Week-level performance drift:

Repeated cycles without full restoration produce slight declines in maximal output. Recovery feels incrementally slower.

Month-level adaptation plateau:

Training stimulus fails to generate expected progression. Strength or endurance plateaus despite consistent effort. Cognitive output ceiling lowers subtly.

Long-term ceiling reduction:

Maximal capacity resets downward. What was previously moderate intensity now feels demanding. The individual stabilizes at a lower output tier.

Importantly, acute fatigue differs from cumulative capacity reduction. Acute fatigue follows unusually high demand or short-term sleep disruption and resolves with recovery. Cumulative capacity reduction reflects allocation reprioritization over time. Rest days may restore transient fatigue but do not restore prior ceiling if marginal availability persists.

Consider an athlete maintaining consistent timing restriction while training moderately and consuming proportionate intake. Performance metrics rise gradually. Recovery between sessions is predictable. Body weight remains stable. Oscillation remains intact. No ceiling compression occurs.

Now consider a similar athlete increasing training volume while maintaining identical intake within the same feeding window. Early weeks feel manageable. By mid-cycle, top-end output drifts downward. Perceived exertion increases for the same workload. Body weight remains unchanged due to subtle reductions in spontaneous movement. Plateau emerges.

The training program appears less effective, yet the underlying variable is cumulative resource mismatch.

Cognitive narrowing can occur even when physical workload remains constant. An individual engaged in high cognitive demand while practicing timing restriction may experience steady daily energy but reduced creative capacity or sustained analytical depth. The difference between baseline functioning and maximal throughput becomes apparent only under prolonged mental strain.

Performance decline often precedes overt metabolic signals because allocation shifts protect essential processes first. Body weight may remain stable due to compensatory adjustments in expenditure. Visible structural markers lag behind functional output changes. The system trims discretionary output quietly before altering core maintenance.

Plateau can mask resource reprioritization. A stable plateau in training performance may appear neutral. However, if prior trajectory indicated upward adaptation, the plateau may represent a lowered ceiling relative to potential. The individual can maintain but cannot progress. Without overt fatigue or weight loss, the shift is easily overlooked.

The distinction between "can function" and "can progress" becomes central. Functioning indicates preserved baseline capacity. Progression indicates surplus allocation toward adaptation. Under marginal availability, functioning is preserved longer than progression.

Reduced adaptation to training stimulus is another early marker. Muscle protein synthesis and mitochondrial adaptation require surplus energy beyond maintenance. When intake matches only baseline demands, adaptation slows. Training still occurs. Improvement stalls.

Slower recovery kinetics reinforce this pattern. Minor muscle soreness persists longer. Sleep quality may remain adequate, yet restoration feels incomplete. These signals accumulate gradually.

Hidden conservation does not imply imminent breakdown. It reflects strategic reprioritization. The organism defers optional output to maintain core stability. When marginal availability continues, the lowered ceiling becomes the new equilibrium.

In contexts where timing restriction aligns with adequate restoration, performance remains robust. In contexts where marginal availability persists across cycles, output decline reveals allocation shift before body composition or overt metabolic markers change.

Performance capacity is therefore the earliest visible marker of allocation reprioritization under sustained marginal availability, signaling subtle shifts in resource distribution before structural breakdown becomes apparent.

Performance capacity also contracts across domains. Physical output and cognitive throughput do not narrow independently. When resource availability trends marginal, subtle reductions in training output can coincide with diminished cognitive resilience. The organism preserves baseline functioning across both domains, but the upper range of capacity in each narrows in parallel. Because reductions occur gradually and proportionally, they may escape detection when evaluated in isolation.

Capacity contraction often stabilizes into a new baseline without conscious recognition. After several months of plateau, the reduced ceiling becomes normalized. Workloads are adjusted downward. Training intensity is unconsciously modulated. Cognitive tasks are distributed differently. Adaptation inertia develops: the system now operates comfortably at a lower maximum because allocation has reprioritized consistently across time.

This inertia explains why restoration after prolonged marginal availability does not immediately restore prior capacity. Once allocation has stabilized at a lower discretionary tier, re-expansion requires sustained proportionate availability across cycles. The narrowing was gradual; widening follows similar temporal rules.

Another distinguishing feature of allocation-driven capacity reduction is reduced responsiveness to stimulus. Training intensity that once produced measurable adaptation now maintains the status quo. Cognitive challenge that once sharpened focus now feels neutral. The system is not incapable of response; it is operating within a tightened discretionary margin.

This differs from acute overreaching. Acute overreaching presents as temporary suppression of output followed by rebound when recovery is provided. Allocation-driven reduction persists despite short rest periods because the underlying proportion between mobilization and restoration remains unchanged. Day-level recovery cannot override month-level allocation shift.

Perceived energy smoothing can reinforce misinterpretation. An individual may report stable fasting comfort and stable body weight while maximal output remains suppressed. The absence of overt fatigue is interpreted as sufficiency. In reality, the system has redistributed resources conservatively. Stability at baseline masks contraction at the ceiling.

Performance capacity therefore functions as an early and sensitive indicator not because it is fragile, but because it is optional. Essential systems are insulated. Discretionary output absorbs constraint first. When intake proportion fully supports demand, discretionary capacity expands. When proportion trends marginal, discretionary capacity contracts quietly.

Across repeated cycles, this contraction can accumulate until a lower-output equilibrium is established. The individual remains functional. However, the potential range has narrowed relative to prior state.

Performance capacity reveals allocation reprioritization before structural breakdown becomes visible because it occupies the surplus tier of the hierarchy. It reflects not whether the organism can survive, but whether it can adapt, progress, and sustain maximal output under demand.

Small mismatches between energy demand and restoration rarely present as immediate failure. They accumulate. The organism compensates at each stage, smoothing short-term instability while gradually adjusting long-term capacity. Over extended horizons, this accumulation produces capacity drift—a downward recalibration of maximal output that occurs without overt disruption.

Capacity drift is architectural rather than episodic. It does not emerge from a single demanding week or an isolated phase of restriction. It develops through repeated cycles in which restoration slightly underperforms mobilization. Each cycle appears manageable. The cumulative effect becomes visible only across longer time scales.

Multi-layer time modeling clarifies this process.

Day level:

Minor under-restoration is absorbed. Stored substrates compensate. Subjective energy remains steady. Performance appears intact.

Week level:

Subtle drift begins. Recovery between high-output efforts lengthens slightly. Motivation fluctuates modestly. These changes are often attributed to normal variability.

Month level:

Adaptation to stimulus slows. Gains plateau. Cognitive throughput narrows under prolonged demand. Spontaneous movement decreases slightly without conscious intention. The organism has begun reallocating discretionary output.

Season level:

The prior performance ceiling becomes less accessible. What once felt moderate now requires deliberate effort. The new level feels stable because it is internally coherent, even though it is lower than previous capacity.

Year level:

The recalibrated ceiling is normalized. The earlier tier of capacity is remembered but no longer expected. Stability is perceived. Drift has become baseline.

Structural margin refers to surplus capacity beyond immediate adequacy. It is the buffer that allows an organism not only to maintain function but to expand, adapt, and absorb volatility without loss of coherence. Adequacy preserves baseline. Surplus preserves potential.

The distinction between adequacy and surplus is subtle but consequential. Adequacy means restoration meets present demand closely enough to prevent overt decline. Surplus means restoration exceeds immediate demand sufficiently to permit adaptation, growth, and resilience under future stressors. Both states may feel stable in the short term. Their long-horizon trajectories differ.

Structural margin functions as a buffer against volatility. When unexpected workload increases, sleep compresses temporarily, or psychological demand intensifies, preserved margin absorbs the perturbation. Output remains near baseline. Recovery remains efficient. Adaptation continues. Without margin, similar perturbations compress capacity quickly.

Margin is a prerequisite for growth. Training stimulus, cognitive challenge, and stress adaptation require energy beyond maintenance. Without surplus proportion sustained across cycles, the system allocates resources toward preservation rather than expansion. Maintenance-level equilibrium can feel stable, yet growth responsiveness declines.

Capacity elasticity reflects the presence of margin. Elastic systems stretch under load and return to prior baseline without lasting contraction. Fragile systems maintain stability under narrow conditions but contract quickly under variation. Elasticity signals surplus integration; fragility signals margin contraction.

Consider an example of preserved structural margin across years. An individual practices consistent timing restriction while maintaining restoration proportionate not only to current workload but with periodic phases of lower demand. Across seasons, training volume fluctuates. During high-volume periods, output remains robust. During lower-volume phases, adaptation continues modestly. Sleep disruption during travel does not meaningfully reduce performance. Variability tolerance reveals preserved margin.

Contrast this with stable maintenance without surplus. An individual maintains steady output year after year without overt decline. Body weight remains stable. Daily function is smooth. However, performance metrics plateau and remain static. Increases in workload produce disproportionate fatigue. Adaptation responsiveness is minimal. Stability is preserved, yet elasticity is absent. The system maintains but does not expand.

The architectural difference between these states lies in long-horizon proportion. In the first, restoration dominance periodically exceeds demand, reinforcing surplus. In the second, restoration closely matches demand without exceeding it. Both appear stable in day-to-day life. Only under stress or opportunity for growth does divergence become visible.

Variability tolerance serves as a marker of preserved margin. An elastic system tolerates irregular meal timing during travel without loss of appetite rhythm. It absorbs a week of intensified workload without performance collapse. It sustains cognitive throughput during prolonged projects without extended recovery lag. These responses indicate surplus proportion across cycles.

Fragile stability, by contrast, requires strict continuity. Minor deviations in sleep or workload produce disproportionate strain. Performance recovers slowly. Cognitive resilience narrows. The system is balanced at maintenance threshold without buffer.

Long-horizon capacity preservation is less about precision and more about proportion dominance. When restoration recurrently exceeds mobilization across cycles, structural margin widens. When restoration only narrowly meets mobilization, stability persists but potential contracts gradually.

Timing structure remains secondary to proportion. A compressed window with sustained surplus preserves margin. A broad window with maintenance-level adequacy may not. Architecture follows proportion, not clock.

Structural margin is therefore the defining variable separating stable maintenance from expandable capacity. It is built through sustained surplus integration across cycles and revealed through elasticity under variation. Without it, systems maintain coherence but lose optionality. With it, systems absorb volatility and expand ceiling over time.

Long-horizon capacity preservation is determined by sustained surplus proportion across cycles, shaping structural margin and elasticity beyond the influence of timing structure alone.

Cortisol, Sleep, and Recovery Integrity

A controlled structure is not synonymous with a robust system. Structure refers to patterned regularity—predictable timing, consistent distribution, repeated cycles. Robustness refers to the capacity to absorb disturbance without losing functional ceiling or requiring disproportionate recovery. The two often coexist, but they are not identical.

A system can appear stable under narrow conditions yet destabilize when those conditions shift. Robustness is revealed not by baseline smoothness, but by response to perturbation.

Variability functions as a stress test of architecture. Travel alters meal timing and sleep duration. Illness disrupts appetite and activity. Workload spikes compress recovery. These perturbations expose whether stability rests on precision or on margin.

An elastic system absorbs disturbance with limited ceiling loss. Output may dip temporarily, but recovery kinetics are rapid. Appetite realigns. Energy stabilizes without prolonged drift. Elasticity indicates structural tolerance bands wide enough to accommodate deviation.

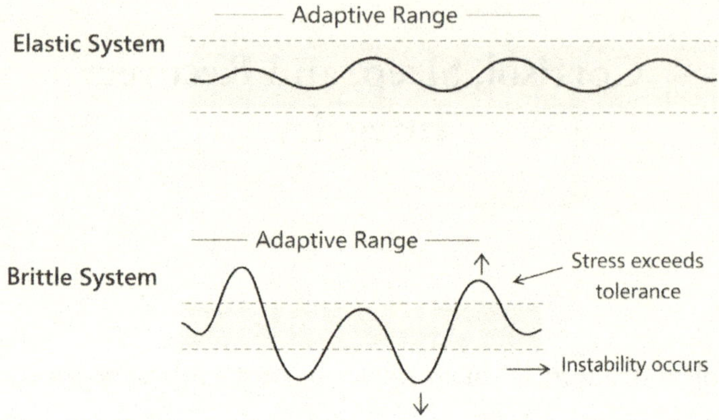

Figure 1 — Elastic vs Brittle Adaptive Systems

A brittle system maintains equilibrium only within narrow parameters. Minor deviation produces disproportionate destabilization. Recovery is slow. Ceiling loss persists beyond the perturbation window. Brittleness signals that stability depends on tight control rather than on integrated buffer.

Acute disruption differs from structural fragility. An acute disruption—such as a short illness or a single night of poor sleep—temporarily suppresses output in nearly any system. Fragility becomes evident when suppression extends disproportionately beyond the disturbance or when repeated small perturbations produce compounding loss.

Robustness can be modeled across common perturbations.

Travel:

Time-zone shifts alter circadian cues and feeding windows. An elastic system may experience temporary appetite displacement but regains rhythm within days. Performance returns to baseline quickly. A brittle system may exhibit prolonged sleep disruption, appetite volatility, and reduced output that persists after routine resumes.

Illness:

Appetite and intake often decrease transiently. Elastic systems restore intake and performance with limited lag. Brittle systems experience prolonged appetite suppression and delayed return of capacity.

Sleep disruption:

One or two shortened nights temporarily reduce performance. In a robust architecture, recovery sleep restores ceiling rapidly. In a brittle architecture, performance drift continues even after sleep normalizes.

Workload spikes:

Short-term increases in demand are absorbed by elastic systems with temporary strain but preserved long-term trajectory. Brittle systems display plateau or regression after modest spikes.

Recovery kinetics serve as a marker of robustness. The speed with which capacity returns to baseline after perturbation reveals margin. Rapid recovery indicates surplus proportion integrated across prior cycles. Slow recovery indicates limited buffer.

Redundancy contributes to robustness. Redundancy does not imply inefficiency; it implies overlapping capacity. Multiple pathways support output. Muscle mass, sleep integrity, cognitive reserves, and nutrient stores collectively create redundancy. When one variable is strained, others compensate.

Over-controlled systems often lack redundancy. Precision-dependent stability—where timing, distribution, and routine must remain exact—can mask fragility. Such systems appear optimized but function within narrow tolerance bands. When deviation occurs, destabilization follows because little buffer exists.

Consider an elastic system maintaining consistent timing structure while integrating sufficient margin. During a week of travel with altered meal timing and shortened sleep, appetite rhythm shifts temporarily.

Training output decreases modestly but rebounds within days of routine resumption. No long-term ceiling contraction occurs. Variability is absorbed.

Contrast this with a brittle system reliant on tight control. A one-hour shift in meal timing produces disproportionate hunger volatility. Sleep disruption extends for weeks after travel. Training plateau persists despite resumption of the normal schedule. The perturbation reveals a narrow equilibrium band.

Precision-dependent stability may appear disciplined and consistent. Margin-based stability appears flexible. The former requires maintenance of exact conditions. The latter tolerates deviation without significant cost.

Fragility can be masked by precision. When the environment remains controlled, brittle systems appear stable. Only perturbation reveals limited tolerance. Elastic systems reveal resilience even when routine shifts.

Structural tolerance bands define how much deviation can occur without ceiling loss. Wider bands reflect integrated margin across cycles. Narrow bands reflect maintenance-level equilibrium without surplus.

Recovery speed differences illustrate this contrast. Two individuals experience an identical workload spike. One returns to prior performance baseline within days. The other requires weeks to regain capacity despite resuming routine. The divergence reflects robustness, not effort.

Stability and adaptability are distinct properties. Stability refers to maintenance under consistent conditions. Adaptability refers to preservation of function under changing conditions. Robust systems maintain both. Brittle systems maintain stability only under narrow constraints.

Rigid precision may create the appearance of control, but control without buffer reduces robustness. Systems that require exact adherence to maintain baseline often lack the integrated margin needed to absorb variation.

Robustness emerges from integrated margin and variability tolerance accumulated across repeated cycles. It is not the product of rigid control, but of structural resilience that allows perturbation without enduring ceiling loss.

Robustness is therefore a function of integrated margin and variability tolerance rather than precise control within narrow structural boundaries.

Metabolic stability is thus defined not by the absence of fluctuation, but by preservation of capacity and trajectory under variability—demonstrating elasticity rather than rigid equilibrium.

Control and resilience are frequently conflated. Both can produce smooth daily output. Both can create the appearance of stability. Their underlying architectures differ.

Control-based stability relies on constraint. Inputs are tightly regulated. Timing is exact. Environmental conditions are kept consistent. Deviation is minimized. Under these static conditions, output appears stable. The system performs predictably because variables are constrained within narrow parameters.

Resilience-based stability relies on integration. Inputs may vary. Timing may shift modestly. Environmental conditions fluctuate. Despite this variability, output remains within functional range. The system performs predictably not because inputs are fixed, but because tolerance bands are wide.

Precision-dependent equilibrium emerges when stability requires exact inputs. Feeding windows must begin and end at specific times. Sleep must occur within narrow duration bands. Workload must remain within predictable limits. Within this equilibrium band, performance appears smooth. Outside it, destabilization occurs.

The mechanics of narrow tolerance bands are subtle. When variability is minimized for extended periods, the system becomes optimized for that specific configuration. Efficiency improves within those constraints.

However, optimization often trades off with robustness. As systems specialize for narrow inputs, flexibility may compress.

Efficiency and robustness exist in tension. A system engineered for maximal efficiency under static conditions may reduce redundancy. Redundancy—overlapping capacity across domains—provides buffer. Removing redundancy increases efficiency but narrows tolerance.

Over-control can compress adaptive bandwidth by eliminating small perturbations that would otherwise rehearse recovery. Without manageable variability, tolerance bands may shrink silently. The system remains stable only as long as conditions remain precise.

Consider an example of precision-dependent stability. An individual maintains exact feeding windows, consistent sleep timing, and uniform workload. Performance remains stable under these conditions. During a short trip requiring a two-hour shift in meal timing and modest sleep compression, appetite volatility increases markedly. Sleep quality declines for several nights. Training output regresses. The deviation was small; the destabilization was disproportionate. Stability depended on environmental precision rather than internal elasticity.

Contrast this with a flexible system. Another individual maintains similar baseline timing but tolerates modest shifts periodically due to a variable schedule. During identical travel conditions, appetite shifts temporarily but realigns within days. Performance dips briefly but rebounds quickly. Sleep stabilizes without extended lag. The same perturbation reveals structural resilience rather than fragility.

The contrast lies not in baseline smoothness, but in response to deviation.

Environmental control can mimic resilience. When the environment is tightly managed, performance variability is minimized. Yet this stability is externally regulated. Remove environmental constraints and underlying fragility becomes visible.

Structural resilience, by contrast, is internally integrated. It persists despite environmental shifts. The system carries its stability with it rather than borrowing it from controlled conditions.

Over-optimization further illustrates this distinction. A system tuned aggressively for narrow performance metrics—precise timing, minimal variability, maximal efficiency—may initially show improved output. However, tolerance for deviation declines. Small changes in input create disproportionate responses because adaptive range has compressed.

An escalation attempt can expose narrow tolerance. Suppose an individual shortens feeding windows incrementally in pursuit of marginal efficiency gains. Within the original window, stability was preserved. With further compression, performance becomes more sensitive to minor workload fluctuations. Recovery slows after small stressors. The intensification appears logical within an optimization framework, yet it reveals limited elasticity.

Latent instability often remains hidden under routine. Only when routine fails does the structural weakness become evident. A missed meal, unexpected workload spike, or minor illness functions as a diagnostic perturbation. If output collapses or recovery lags excessively, stability was dependent on precision.

Variability avoidance reduces rehearsal of recovery. Systems that avoid deviation entirely may lose capacity to absorb it. By contrast, systems exposed to moderate variability develop familiarity with perturbation and restoration cycles.

Control-based systems often rely on external regulation: fixed schedules, strict timing, tightly managed inputs. Resilient systems rely on internal integration: preserved margin, wide tolerance bands, and efficient recovery.

Ceiling loss under small deviation reveals fragile equilibrium. If maximal output contracts significantly after minor perturbation, tolerance bands are narrow. If ceiling returns quickly, tolerance bands are wide.

True stability must therefore be evaluated under dynamic conditions rather than static ones. Static smoothness does not guarantee preserved capacity. Dynamic resilience—maintenance of trajectory under variability—signals integrated architecture.

Externally enforced precision can produce short-term steadiness. Internally integrated resilience produces long-term stability. The difference becomes visible only when precision fails.

An elastic envelope model captures this distinction. An envelope describes the range of outputs the system can produce and recover from without losing ceiling. A narrow envelope permits stability only under limited inputs. A wide envelope allows stability under varied inputs. Elasticity refers to the ability to stretch temporarily under demand and return without enduring contraction.

This elasticity is cross-domain. Physical output can remain stable even when cognitive load increases if recovery calibration remains efficient. Cognitive throughput can remain stable during travel if sleep disruption is temporary and integrated. Environmental unpredictability does not have to become physiological volatility when the envelope is wide enough.

Cross-domain coherence means that perturbations in one domain do not automatically cascade into dysfunction in another. A workload spike may reduce training output temporarily without collapsing appetite rhythm or sleep continuity. A short sleep disruption may blunt performance briefly without shifting baseline for weeks. The system remains integrated rather than fragmented.

Escalation testing functions as a diagnostic, not a performance pursuit. When demand rises—longer work hours, higher training load, tighter schedules—the system reveals whether its stability is conditional or portable. If small increases in demand produce disproportionate ceiling loss or prolonged recovery lag, tolerance bands are narrow. If capacity remains accessible and recovery is proportionate, the architecture is robust.

Portable stability across changing environments illustrates this maturity. Consider an individual whose schedule varies seasonally: winter involves long work hours and minimal travel; summer involves travel and later meals; autumn increases training volume. Across these shifts, baseline rhythm changes modestly, but the ceiling remains available. Performance may dip temporarily during travel, then return rapidly. Appetite aligns without prolonged volatility. Sleep compresses during peak workload, yet recovery stabilizes once workload normalizes without lingering drift. Stability is carried across contexts.

Context-bound stability looks similar under controlled conditions but fails portability tests. Another individual maintains near-perfect stability in a fixed routine. When a new project increases cognitive demand and shifts meal timing by two hours, sleep fragments for weeks and training performance declines persistently. The daily structure had been stable; the architecture was narrow. Stability depended on the environment remaining unchanged.

Recovery integration is the reinforcement mechanism that widens tolerance over time. When perturbations are followed by sufficient restoration, the system learns that disturbance is survivable and bounded. This does not require constant variation; it requires that variation, when it occurs, is integrated rather than compounded. Each completed perturbation–recovery cycle functions as architectural strengthening. Over time, tolerance bands widen and responses become more proportional.

A separate example clarifies this strengthening. An individual experiences intermittent periods of high occupational demand several times each year. Early on, each period produces prolonged performance lag. Over time, as recovery phases are consistently integrated afterward, the lag shortens. The system becomes less reactive and more proportional. The perturbations have not disappeared; the response has matured.

Fasting structures must support this variability competence to remain stable over the long horizon. A timing structure that requires exact conditions to function—precise windows that cannot flex, rigid intake placement that cannot absorb travel or workload change—encourages environmental dependency. It may create short-term smoothness at the cost of portability. A timing structure that remains coherent through modest variability contributes to envelope expansion. The structure becomes part of the system's architecture rather than an external constraint that the environment must protect.

Stability under escalation, not just under maintenance, distinguishes mature systems. Maintenance stability is the ability to keep baseline consistent when life is stable. Escalation stability is the ability to preserve ceiling and trajectory when demands rise. The latter is the more revealing test because it exposes whether stability is built on internal integration or external control.

This is not optimization language. It is architectural evaluation. Stability is measured by capacity preservation and recovery proportionality under changing conditions, not by how narrow the routine can be made.

Mature metabolic systems are characterized by an expandable envelope: the ability to tolerate greater variability and higher demand without losing coherence. The envelope expands through integrated cycles of perturbation and recovery, supported by margin and wide tolerance bands. Conditional stability remains narrow because it avoids perturbation rather than integrating it.

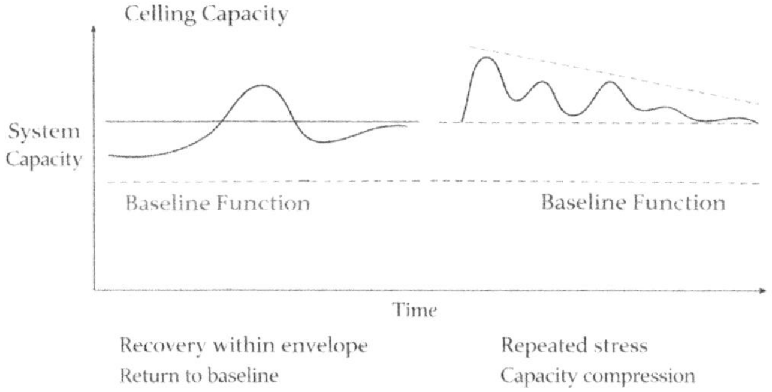

Figure 2 — Capacity Envelope and Recovery Return

Variability-competent architecture expresses itself across multiple temporal layers. Day-level fluctuation is routine. Week-level compression may occur during elevated demand. Season-level change tests whether the envelope contracts or maintains width. Year-level trajectory reveals whether capacity remains expandable or stabilizes at a constrained tier. Portability is proven when envelope width persists across these scales rather than resetting downward after each phase of intensity.

Maintenance competence and expansion competence are not identical. A system may preserve baseline functioning indefinitely under predictable load yet resist upward adjustment when opportunity arises. Expansion competence reflects retained elasticity—the ability to increase demand without disproportionate strain or prolonged recalibration. Variability-competent systems maintain both: they protect baseline and preserve the option to expand.

Compound escalation is the decisive diagnostic. When demand increases simultaneously across domains—longer work hours during intensified training, compressed sleep during travel, environmental unpredictability layered onto cognitive load—the envelope is tested under real-world complexity. Conditional systems often display ceiling compression under such stacking. Integrated systems experience temporary narrowing but restore full width once the perturbation resolves.

Portability across life phases further clarifies architectural maturity. As context evolves—career shifts, aging, family demands, travel frequency—the externally controlled variables inevitably change. Stability that depends on static conditions erodes gradually under these transitions. Stability grounded in integrated margin and adaptive range persists because it is internally maintained rather than environmentally protected.

Conditional stability narrows tolerance bands through dependency. Intrinsic stability widens tolerance bands through integration. The former requires preservation of circumstance. The latter survives circumstance.

Fasting structures participate in this architecture as organizing elements, not as stability generators in isolation. When timing structures reinforce envelope width—allowing modest variability without destabilization—they integrate into resilience. When they require environmental protection to remain intact, they narrow portability. The structure should serve the system's elasticity, not replace it.

Integrated stability therefore includes oscillation tolerance, escalation tolerance, portability across contexts, and preservation of ceiling under compound variability. It is less concerned with eliminating fluctuation than with preserving capacity through it.

Metabolic stability, viewed architecturally, is variability-competent capacity preserved across escalation and environmental change—an expandable envelope maintained through integrated recovery and cross-domain coherence rather than rigid equilibrium enforced by precise control.

Caloric Deficit vs Timing Illusion

Energy balance is often discussed as a daily number. In biological systems, it functions more accurately as long-horizon accounting. Tissue change reflects proportion across repeated cycles rather than substrate use within isolated hours.

A fasting interval increases fat oxidation during that interval. This is a normal metabolic shift. When intake is absent, circulating insulin declines, glycogen availability decreases, and reliance on stored substrate increases. Fatty acids contribute more significantly to energy production. This acute oxidation is visible in respiratory exchange measurements and fuel utilization data.

Acute oxidation, however, does not equal net tissue loss.

Mobilization refers to the release and oxidation of stored substrate during energy demand. Depletion refers to sustained reduction in stored tissue mass across time. Mobilization occurs daily, even in individuals who gain weight over months. Depletion requires that mobilization consistently exceeds restoration across extended cycles. Structural change occurs only when restoration fails to match mobilization across repeated cycles.

The distinction between substrate switching and energy balance becomes central here. Substrate switching describes which fuel source is used at a given moment. Energy balance describes whether total intake matches or diverges from total expenditure across days and weeks. One can increase fat oxidation transiently without altering net fat mass if restoration later matches mobilization.

Partitioning must also be distinguished from balance. During fasting intervals, a higher proportion of energy may derive from fat. During feeding, a portion of intake may be directed toward glycogen repletion before fat storage occurs. Partitioning determines which substrates are used at a given moment. Balance determines whether total stored energy mass changes.

Consider intra-day fat oxidation during a prolonged fasting interval. During the fasting phase, fat stores supply energy. Later, during the feeding window, intake may restore glycogen and contribute to fat storage if total energy exceeds expenditure for the day. Over 24 hours, the mobilization–restoration cycle may balance out. Fat oxidation occurred. Net fat mass remained unchanged.

This dynamic illustrates why oxidation during fasting does not guarantee fat loss. Structural tissue change requires a sustained proportion mismatch in which total energy intake remains below total expenditure across repeated cycles. The body integrates over time.

Day-level deficit can be erased by week-level compensation. An individual may create a modest deficit during weekdays through timing restriction, only to increase intake during weekends. Weekly energy balance determines net tissue change more reliably than daily oscillation.

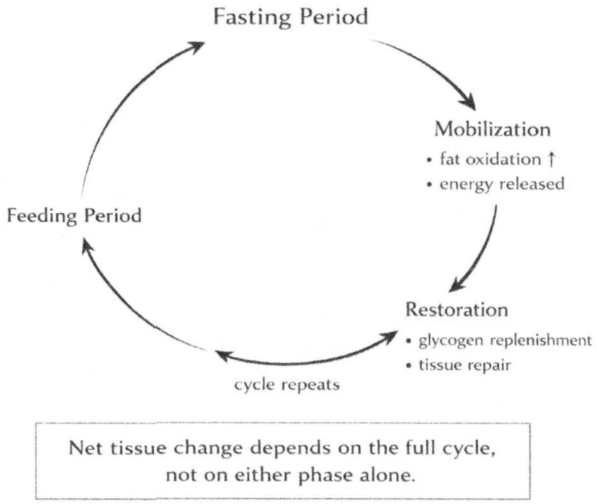

Figure 3 — Mobilization and Restoration Across a Feeding Cycle

Behavioral containment—the use of a feeding window to limit eating opportunities—can reduce intake for some individuals. For others, appetite may increase within the window, leading to equal or greater total intake. The timing structure does not inherently create deficit. It reorganizes opportunity.

A clear example illustrates fasting without net deficit. An individual consumes two large meals within a six-hour window. During the fasting interval, fat oxidation rises. During the feeding window, total intake matches expenditure for the day. Body weight remains stable over months. Fat oxidation occurs daily. Net fat mass does not decline.

Conversely, modest deficit can occur without fasting. An individual eats three meals distributed across twelve hours but consumes slightly less total energy than expended each day. Over weeks, body fat decreases gradually despite frequent feeding. Substrate switching may be less pronounced during the day, yet net balance drives structural change.

The contrast between visible oxidation and structural fat loss clarifies this distinction. Visible oxidation refers to measured substrate use at a given time. Structural loss refers to cumulative reduction in adipose tissue. The former fluctuates hourly. The latter reflects long-horizon proportion.

Compensation further complicates intra-day interpretation. A person may consume no calories until afternoon, increasing fat oxidation during morning hours. Later, hunger intensifies, leading to larger meals. If those meals fully compensate for earlier abstention, the net 24-hour energy balance may equal maintenance. The fasting interval created mobilization but not depletion.

Metabolic smoothing can mask this dynamic. Individuals may feel steady energy across fasting intervals and interpret this stability as deficit. Yet smoothing reflects improved handling of substrate switching rather than confirmation of negative balance. Appetite and intake determine restoration.

Mobilization–restoration modeling clarifies structural change. During fasting hours, mobilization predominates. During feeding hours, restoration predominates. If restoration equals mobilization across cycles, tissue mass remains stable. If mobilization modestly exceeds restoration across repeated cycles, depletion occurs gradually. The time horizon matters.

The confusion comes from mixing hour-level fuel choice with week-level accounting. Deficit must be sustained across days and weeks to alter stored energy mass. Timing restriction can create such mismatch if intake remains proportionately lower than expenditure. It can also coexist with maintenance or surplus if intake compensates.

Energy balance must be understood across layered time scales. Hour-level substrate use shifts rapidly. Day-level balance reflects aggregate intake and expenditure. Week-level balance reveals sustained proportion. Month-level balance determines structural tissue change. Confusion arises when hour-level oxidation is mistaken for week-level deficit.

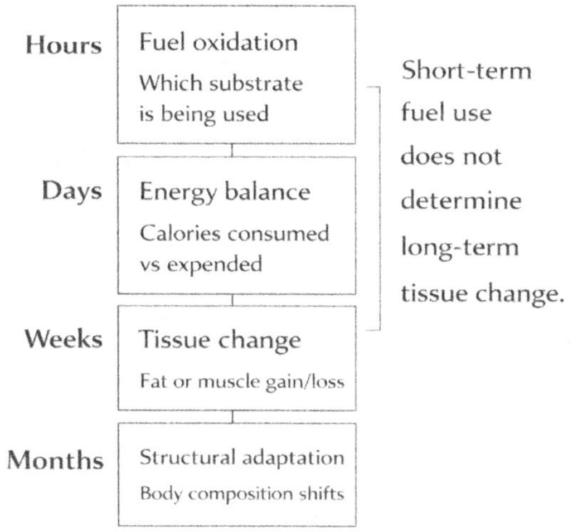

Figure 4 — Energy Balance Operates Across Multiple Time Scales

Energy flux symmetry further clarifies the illusion. During fasting, fat flux increases outward from adipose tissue. During feeding, flux reverses inward if intake supplies excess energy. Both fluxes can be large while net balance remains neutral. High turnover does not equal net loss unless mobilization exceeds restoration across cycles. Structural change requires asymmetry across the full cycle.

Short-horizon perception amplifies this misunderstanding. The experience of using stored fuel feels meaningful because it is metabolically distinct. However, the body does not preserve a memory of oxidation hours; it integrates total balance. Repeated oxidation that is later offset by equivalent restoration produces turnover without depletion.

Compensation elasticity explains why containment does not automatically equal deficit. Some individuals compress intake without increasing density, resulting in lower total intake. Others unconsciously increase meal size, caloric density, or post-fast consumption. The feeding window becomes denser even if shorter. Structural deficit depends on total intake relative to expenditure, not on the duration of eating opportunity.

Escalation modeling illustrates this distinction. A person may extend fasting duration incrementally, increasing the hours of fat oxidation. If intake later expands proportionally, net balance remains unchanged. Duration increased; deficit did not. Only when total intake fails to match total expenditure across repeated cycles does structural loss occur.

Deficit dominance must persist across weeks to produce visible tissue change. A small negative balance maintained consistently produces gradual depletion. A large intra-day swing offset by later compensation produces metabolic turnover without net change. The organism integrates across cycles, not across single fasting intervals.

Behavioral containment is therefore a tool, not a mechanism. It may reduce intake for some individuals by limiting opportunity. It may fail for others if compensatory intake increases. The structure modifies behavior probability, not energy law.

Containment changes opportunity; it does not guarantee deficit. Oxidation during fasting is real. Structural depletion is conditional. Only sustained proportion mismatch across repeated cycles alters stored mass.

A feeding window can compress time without compressing intake. Hours disappear; energy does not necessarily follow. The clock tightens, meals cluster, and the daily structure appears leaner. Yet inside that shortened span, subtle expansions often unfold.

When morning intake is removed, the first meal of the day rarely remains unchanged. Hunger accumulated during the fasting interval expresses itself through size, pace, and selection. Portions increase slightly. Energy-dense components move closer to the center of the meal. What had been a moderate portion becomes, almost imperceptibly, a larger one. The shift rarely announces itself; it feels proportional to the delay.

Inside a compressed window, density often rises. Two meals can quietly carry the weight of three. A lunch that once followed breakfast may now absorb both appetites. A dinner that previously concluded the day may expand to secure satiety against the coming fast. Each adjustment is small. The aggregate effect restores balance.

Palatability shifts alongside portion size. After extended abstention, highly rewarding foods often feel more compelling. Flavor intensity and caloric concentration become more appealing. Selection drifts subtly toward richer options. The change is rarely dramatic; it is cumulative. What had been a balanced plate gradually tilts toward higher density without overt recognition.

Containment is visible. Reduction is not guaranteed. Limiting eating to certain hours removes grazing opportunities and compresses decision points. For some individuals, that containment translates into lower intake. For others, the same structure reorganizes appetite into fewer but larger events. Time shrinks; energy redistributes.

The first meal after fasting often carries a disproportionate caloric load. What might have been distributed across breakfast and lunch consolidates into a single episode. Satiety signals may lag behind rapid consumption, especially when hunger is amplified by anticipation. The meal ends when fullness becomes clear rather than when adequacy is reached. The difference between those two points can be small but consistent.

These changes are rarely intentional. They unfold through alignment between hunger intensity and meal composition. The body seeks equilibrium. If intake is deferred, it tends to be restored.

Across the week, patterns further reshape balance. An individual may maintain disciplined containment from Monday through Friday, eating within a narrow window and feeling in control of structure. During those days, intake drifts modestly downward. By Friday evening, accumulated appetite and social engagement expand opportunity. Saturday meals lengthen. Portions increase. Dessert appears where it had been absent. Sunday includes a late brunch and an extended dinner. By week's end, the modest weekday deficit dissolves into neutrality.

The weekday structure remains intact. The feeding window was respected. Yet the weekly arc absorbs the difference.

In another case, the shift is quieter. An individual eliminates breakfast and feels steady through the morning. Lunch grows slightly larger than before, but the change feels justified by delayed eating. Dinner appears similar in size, though small additions—an extra serving, a caloric beverage, a more generous portion of starch—creep in. None of these changes seem consequential in isolation. Over weeks, they equal the energy once consumed at breakfast.

Compensation elasticity differs between individuals. Some experience appetite that dampens with repetition, allowing total intake to remain modestly lower without strain. Others experience appetite that intensifies proportionally to restriction, restoring prior intake levels. The feeding window does not dictate which response occurs.

Containment can therefore be mistaken for reduction. The schedule is tighter. The number of meals is smaller. The visible markers of restraint are present. But true reduction requires sustained divergence between intake and expenditure. Containment merely narrows opportunity. Whether opportunity translates into lower total intake depends on compensation dynamics.

The contrast becomes clearer when observing two individuals using identical timing. One maintains moderate meal size within the window and does not substantially increase density. Spontaneous movement remains stable. Weekend intake resembles weekday intake. Over time, body composition shifts modestly. The deficit persists because compensation remains incomplete.

The other individual compresses eating hours but responds with larger meals and richer food choices. Weekend intake expands. Activity declines slightly. Body composition remains unchanged. The timing structure is identical; the adaptive response differs.

There is also the phenomenon of earned flexibility. After hours of abstention, the meal that follows can feel deserved. The perception is subtle and rarely articulated. It manifests as slightly more generous plating or the inclusion of an energy-dense option that might not have appeared under distributed eating. The shift is incremental, not indulgent. Yet repeated increments restore balance.

Day-level deficit can dissolve into week-level neutrality without dramatic episodes. A modest daily shortfall of intake relative to expenditure may be erased by a single larger social meal. The arithmetic unfolds quietly. The person continues fasting consistently and observes no structural change in timing. The energy system, however, has recalibrated.

Compensation also operates through smoothing. If intake is lower on one day, hunger may intensify the next. Intake increases slightly. Over several days, balance reasserts itself. The organism resists sustained divergence from equilibrium unless mismatch persists across cycles.

This does not render timing ineffective. It clarifies its role. Timing shapes opportunity and appetite rhythm. It does not suspend adaptive recalibration. For some individuals, the compressed structure reduces intake enough to maintain negative proportion across weeks. For others, appetite, density, social context, and output adjustments converge to restore prior balance.

The distinction between containment and reduction defines the difference between structural change and structural preservation. Containment narrows when eating occurs. Reduction alters how much energy enters the system across time. Without reduction, tissue mass remains stable even under visible fasting.

Over months, this recalibration can fully neutralize an intended deficit. The feeding window remains constant. The clock continues to guide intake. Yet the net proportion between intake and expenditure returns to maintenance. The deficit erodes not through dramatic reversal but through incremental adaptation.

Compensation—operating through intake density, appetite amplification, spontaneous movement, and social context—functions as adaptive recalibration capable of neutralizing deficit even when feeding timing remains externally unchanged.

Under-Recovery and Capacity Compression

Energy availability is not merely the presence of calories. It is the proportion of incoming energy relative to the demands placed upon the system. When intake aligns comfortably with workload, restoration keeps pace with mobilization. When intake falls modestly below demand for brief periods, the system tolerates the mismatch with minimal structural consequence. When that mismatch becomes sustained—subtle, persistent, and recurrent—the signal shifts.

Low energy availability functions as an environmental message. The body does not interpret numbers; it interprets patterns. A consistent shortfall relative to workload is registered not as discipline but as scarcity. Scarcity need not be dramatic to be meaningful. A mild but repeated gap between restoration and demand conveys a different environment than one of surplus or balance.

The distinction between short-term deficit and sustained marginal availability lies in duration and repetition. A few days of reduced intake within otherwise adequate cycles usually produce little more than transient adjustment. The system mobilizes stored energy, performance dips slightly, and restoration resumes. When marginal availability extends across weeks or months, the signal becomes integrated. The environment appears leaner—not temporarily, but persistently.

Early adaptations are subtle. Resting expenditure may adjust downward modestly. Spontaneous movement may contract slightly. These changes are not necessarily conscious. They represent economization—small reductions in output that preserve essential processes. The system does not abandon function; it reallocates.

Resource-conservation logic is ancient and pragmatic. When availability declines relative to demand, non-essential or discretionary processes narrow. Performance ceiling compresses before baseline function deteriorates. Adaptation shifts from optimization toward preservation. The objective becomes sustainability under constraint rather than expansion under abundance.

Consider an individual maintaining a mild but sustained deficit relative to workload. Training continues, daily function remains intact, and weight decreases gradually. After months, performance improvements plateau. Recovery between sessions lengthens slightly. Pace remains acceptable but no longer improves. The system has not failed; it has recalibrated to operate within available resources. Output compresses to match restoration capacity.

Plateau is often mistaken for completion of adaptation. In the context of sustained marginal availability, plateau can reflect conservation. The system maintains function but limits expansion. The ceiling compresses quietly. Stability may be interpreted as equilibrium when it actually represents a narrowed range.

Resting-expenditure adjustments are typically small yet meaningful over time. The body economizes through minor reductions in thermogenesis, spontaneous movement, and discretionary activity. None of these changes signal dysfunction; they signal prioritization. Essential processes remain protected.

Recovery kinetics provide another subtle marker. After intense effort, restoration may require longer intervals when availability is marginal. The system conserves by pacing adaptation more cautiously. Growth processes yield to maintenance priorities.

This outer-boundary contraction can persist unnoticed because daily life rarely demands maximal capacity. A moderate training load can be sustained even if prior peak strength has diminished. Work tasks can be completed even if sustained creative depth requires more effort. The system protects essential continuity while trimming discretionary margin.

Adaptive range also narrows under persistent marginal availability. Minor perturbations—an additional training session, a short night of sleep, an unexpected workload spike—produce disproportionate fatigue compared with prior months. Recovery remains possible, but the buffer is thinner. What was once absorbed easily now registers as strain.

Downregulation in this context is not failure. It is proportional response. When the system interprets sustained scarcity relative to demand, it prioritizes maintenance of essential processes. Optional expansion—maximal performance, robust reproductive signaling, rapid adaptation—yields to conservation. The architecture tightens to preserve coherence.

Sustained marginal availability therefore operates as a compression signal that gradually narrows the capacity envelope across systems, prioritizing preservation over expansion without precipitating immediate collapse.

Energy is distributed across tiers. Baseline maintenance—cellular integrity, organ function, and neurological stability—occupies the highest priority. Performance capacity, the ability to produce maximal output beyond baseline requirements, sits lower. Reproductive robustness, growth, and other discretionary processes follow. Under abundant conditions, these tiers operate expansively. Under sustained marginal availability, redistribution occurs.

Consider an individual who trains regularly while maintaining marginal intake relative to workload. Daily energy feels acceptable. Work responsibilities are met. Yet peak sprint times plateau. Strength gains slow. The capacity to push beyond previous limits compresses. The plateau may be attributed to programming or insufficient stimulus variation. The deeper shift lies in allocation. Resources once available for expansion have been redirected toward preservation.

This prioritization logic extends beyond performance. Immune resilience may shift subtly. Minor illnesses can linger slightly longer. Recovery from intense effort may require additional days. These are not dramatic changes; they reflect cautious scaling of non-essential processes under perceived scarcity.

Reproductive signaling serves as environmental readout. When energy availability narrows persistently, the system interprets the environment as less favorable for expansion of future lineage. In some individuals, this may appear as subtle shifts in reproductive robustness—changes in cycle regularity or reduced emphasis on reproductive readiness. These responses are proportional to sustained signals rather than abrupt failures.

Thyroid modulation follows a similar pattern of proportional scaling. When availability contracts relative to demand, metabolic rate adjusts to align expenditure with intake. This adjustment is not an error; it is calibration. It reduces unnecessary expenditure while preserving essential stability.

The narrowing of high-output systems precedes any compromise of baseline survival. Maximal output declines before baseline fails. The body trims capacity at the edges rather than at the core. Because these shifts are gradual, they can be misinterpreted as stagnation unrelated to energy availability.

Preservation of survival precedes expansion by design. Under sustained marginal availability, growth processes yield to stability. Repair remains sufficient for maintenance, while expansion becomes secondary. This reflects prioritization rather than dysfunction.

Optimization requires surplus. Maintenance requires adequacy. Conservation emerges under sustained mismatch. The transition between these states is incremental and adaptive. The system is not failing; it is aligning output with environment.

Within this architecture of energy regulation, certain systems function less as isolated mechanisms and more as interpreters of environment. Thyroid and reproductive signaling operate in this role. They scale and modulate in proportion to availability. Their shifts are often subtle, gradual, and reflective rather than disruptive.

Thyroid signaling acts as a metabolic calibrator. It influences the rate at which energy moves through the system, how readily fuel is oxidized, and how much baseline expenditure is maintained. When availability is ample relative to demand, metabolic rate tends to align with expansion. When availability narrows persistently relative to workload, thyroid output may adjust downward modestly, conserving expenditure without halting function.

Consider an individual maintaining marginal availability over several months while preserving structured eating and consistent activity. Laboratory markers might show small downward shifts in thyroid-related indices, still within normal range. Energy feels steady but not abundant. Performance gains stall despite consistent training stimulus. The modulation reflects calibration, not malfunction. The system is preserving alignment between intake and expenditure.

Reproductive signaling functions as environmental interpretation at another level. It represents permission for expansion—an investment in future energy expenditure through reproduction. When availability signals abundance and resilience, reproductive robustness is reinforced. When availability narrows persistently, signaling may scale down proportionally.

This scaling is rarely dramatic at first. In some individuals, cycle length may vary slightly. Ovulatory timing may shift subtly. In others, libido may fluctuate. These changes often remain within normal biological variation. They reflect environmental readout rather than categorical breakdown.

An example illustrates this proportionality. A physically active individual maintains marginal availability relative to workload. Over time, menstrual cycles become slightly longer and less predictable, though not absent. Daily function remains normal. There is no acute event—only gradual modulation. When restoration increases across subsequent months, cycle regularity returns without intervention. The signaling system responded proportionally to environment and recalibrated when the environment changed.

The body's reluctance to expand under scarcity is logical. Reproduction and high metabolic output require surplus. When surplus is absent across repeated cycles, signaling adapts to conserve. This is not evidence of fragility; it is evidence of environmental sensitivity.

Plateau in performance often accompanies subtle endocrine modulation because both arise from the same proportional logic. When availability remains marginal, expansion slows. Performance stabilizes. Thyroid output scales modestly. Reproductive signaling tempers expansion readiness. These parallel responses reflect systemic coherence rather than independent dysfunction.

Restoration dominance can reverse this modulation gradually. When intake increases proportionately relative to demand across extended cycles, metabolic rate may adjust upward. Reproductive robustness often strengthens. The system does not maintain conservation once the environment shifts; it recalibrates in alignment with sustained signals.

For example, an individual may experience mild cold sensitivity and slightly slower recovery during a period of marginal availability. Training output plateaus. Months later, after restoration increases and workload moderates, warmth perception normalizes and adaptation resumes. No pathology intervened. The system scaled and then rescaled.

Thyroid and reproductive signaling therefore act as environmental indicators. They read sustained patterns of availability and demand, scaling metabolic rate and expansion readiness proportionally. Their modulation reflects adaptive interpretation rather than inherent malfunction.

Performance does not disappear abruptly under sustained marginal availability. It compresses. The outer boundary of what is possible narrows gradually, often without dramatic markers. Daily functioning continues. Training sessions are completed. Cognitive tasks are handled. What changes is the distance between baseline and ceiling.

The performance ceiling represents maximal output under favorable conditions. When energy availability remains proportionate to demand, that ceiling can expand with stimulus. When availability narrows persistently, the ceiling begins to contract. The contraction is subtle at first. A lift that once moved smoothly at a given weight feels slightly heavier. A pace once maintained for intervals requires greater focus. The difference is small, but it repeats.

Recovery margin narrows alongside the ceiling. Margin functions as the buffer between demand and restoration. When margin is wide, a demanding session is followed by rapid restoration. When margin erodes, restoration extends. The individual may still complete the same session, but the recovery window lengthens incrementally.

This extension is not overt exhaustion. It is recalibration. A session that once required a single day of recovery may now require two. A cognitive project that once felt stimulating may leave residual fatigue. Emotional resilience may feel slightly thinner under stress. The system remains functional but less elastic.

Plateau and compression are not identical. Plateau can occur even under adequate availability when stimulus no longer produces adaptation. Compression reflects a reduced capacity envelope regardless of stimulus variation. A plateau under marginal availability may be misread as a programming flaw or insufficient variation. The deeper shift lies in constrained resources rather than design.

An example illustrates this distinction. An athlete follows a structured training plan and experiences steady progress for months. Intake remains marginal relative to increasing workload. Performance gains slow and then halt. The athlete adjusts programming—changing rep schemes, altering volume—but improvement does not resume. The assumption centers on design. The underlying issue is compressed margin. Resources sufficient for maintenance are insufficient for expansion.

High workload amplifies compression. When demands increase while availability remains static, the gap between requirement and restoration widens. Initially, performance may be preserved through mobilization. Over time, outer boundaries narrow. The athlete still trains consistently but no longer responds robustly to stimulus. The ceiling lowers quietly.

Increased workload often reveals hidden compression. An individual may maintain stable output under moderate demand and assume stability is intact. When workload intensifies—a new project, increased training volume—the system struggles disproportionately. Recovery lengthens. Performance declines modestly. The prior stability masked a narrow margin.

Importantly, compression often reveals itself only when compared with prior capacity. In isolation, current performance may appear stable. When examined longitudinally, outer-boundary decline becomes evident. The envelope has shifted inward, preventing the organism from overshooting available resources.

By trimming expansion capacity first, the system maintains coherence under constraint. This protection is intelligent but comes at the cost of elasticity.

Sustained marginal availability therefore acts as a quiet narrowing force on the capacity envelope, compressing performance ceiling and recovery margin gradually rather than precipitating sudden collapse.

The capacity envelope is not fixed. It contracts under sustained marginal availability, and it can widen when the proportion between intake and demand shifts in the opposite direction. This widening is not abrupt. It does not occur in response to a single day of abundance. It unfolds across repeated cycles in which restoration consistently exceeds immediate strain.

When availability becomes sufficient relative to workload, the system begins to interpret the environment differently. Scarcity signals fade. Preservation logic loosens. Expansion permission gradually returns. The outer boundary of performance, previously compressed, begins to extend.

Restoration dominance is the central condition for this re-expansion. A single increase in intake or a brief reduction in workload may produce transient relief but rarely alters structural architecture. Re-expansion requires sustained dominance of restoration across multiple cycles. The system must experience a pattern of adequacy rather than an isolated spike of excess.

As restoration predominates, recovery kinetics shorten and output responsiveness improves. Training stimulus once again produces measurable adaptation. Minor perturbations generate proportionate responses rather than extended lag. The tolerance band widens gradually.

Consider an athlete who has plateaued under sustained marginal availability. Performance gains stalled and recovery lag increased subtly. After several months of proportionately higher restoration and moderated workload, improvement resumes. Weights that once felt heavy regain smoothness. Adaptation again responds to stimulus. The envelope, previously narrowed, widens incrementally.

This widening often appears first in recovery. Sessions that once required extended rest regain predictable restoration intervals. Energy between efforts stabilizes. The system begins allocating resources toward expansion rather than merely preserving baseline.

Reversibility is a defining feature of this architecture. Downregulation under sustained marginal availability is not permanent. It reflects proportional interpretation of environment. When the environment shifts reliably, signaling and performance adjust in parallel.

An individual who experienced persistent plateau, subtle cold sensitivity, and slower adaptation during marginal availability may gradually regain responsiveness after months of improved restoration. Performance resumes upward trajectory. Recovery margins expand. The system recalibrates because the environmental signal has changed.

Re-expansion is therefore cumulative rather than immediate. Just as compression emerges gradually under sustained mismatch, restoration must persist across cycles to reverse the signal. The organism requires repeated confirmation that resources exceed demand.

Capacity is dynamic and proportion-dependent. It can narrow under sustained scarcity and re-expand through repeated restoration across cycles rather than remaining permanently diminished by temporary compression.

When Intermittent Fasting Degrades Stability

Sleep is not an isolated event that occurs at night. It is the visible phase of a circadian architecture that organizes metabolic activity across twenty-four hours. Hormonal rhythms, body-temperature cycles, digestive readiness, cognitive alertness, and appetite signals are coordinated by this internal timing system. Feeding patterns interact with it continuously.

Circadian rhythm functions as a metabolic organizer. During the biological day, alertness and energy mobilization rise. As evening approaches, physiological processes gradually transition toward repair and consolidation. Core temperature falls. Melatonin increases. Digestive efficiency shifts. This orchestration is subtle but consistent.

Feeding timing acts as a powerful cue within this architecture. Regular meal timing reinforces daily rhythm. Irregular or late meals can nudge the system in competing directions. When feeding windows align with natural wakefulness and activity, rhythm coherence tends to be preserved. When feeding windows drift into biological night, conflict can emerge.

A late feeding window illustrates this interaction. An individual who consumes the final meal close to bedtime may experience difficulty initiating sleep. Digestion remains active while melatonin attempts to signal rest. Body temperature may remain elevated. Insulin and nutrient processing overlap with the onset of nocturnal repair. Sleep onset is delayed slightly. The delay may appear minor on a single night, but when repeated across weeks it becomes structural.

Another pattern emerges with early feeding combined with extended fasting into the evening. If the final meal occurs mid-afternoon while workload remains high into the evening, hunger may intensify near bedtime. Elevated appetite signals can interfere with sleep initiation. The body, interpreting prolonged wakefulness and rising hunger, may maintain a mild state of alertness that delays sleep onset.

High workload amplifies these effects. Consider an individual maintaining a compressed feeding window while managing intense cognitive or physical demands late in the day. Stress-related activation rises. If the feeding window ends early, evening hours combine elevated stress with increasing hunger. Sleep onset becomes less stable. Night awakenings may occur more frequently. Recovery margin narrows.

Cortisol rhythm interacts with these patterns. Normally cortisol peaks in the morning and declines through the day. Persistent late-night eating or prolonged late-day stress can blunt this decline. Cortisol remains modestly elevated when it would otherwise taper. The result may not be overt insomnia but lighter or more fragmented sleep.

Appetite rhythm also adapts to feeding timing. When meals are consistently delayed, ghrelin secretion adjusts to anticipate intake. If feeding windows are inconsistent or misaligned with sleep timing, hunger peaks may occur at inconvenient hours. Nighttime hunger can fragment sleep, while early-morning hunger may truncate rest prematurely.

The distinction between occasional disruption and chronic misalignment is central. A late meal on a single evening rarely destabilizes rhythm meaningfully. A week of irregular sleep during travel may produce transient disturbance. Chronic misalignment emerges when feeding timing repeatedly conflicts with circadian cues.

Cumulative circadian drift unfolds quietly. Minor nightly delays in sleep onset accumulate into reduced total sleep duration. Slightly fragmented sleep becomes normalized. Recovery impairment appears as slower training adaptation, reduced cognitive clarity, or subtle mood variability. These shifts are rarely dramatic. They are incremental.

One individual may thrive under a late feeding window if workload is moderate and sleep opportunity is preserved. Another may destabilize under the same window if workload extends late into the evening and recovery opportunity is compressed. The interaction between feeding timing, stress load, and sleep duration determines the outcome.

A stable rhythm displays coherence across domains. Feeding aligns with wakefulness. Hunger subsides before bedtime. Cortisol declines appropriately. Sleep onset becomes predictable. Recovery unfolds efficiently.

In contrast, a drifting rhythm shows small but persistent misalignments. Meals extend into biological night. Hunger peaks at bedtime. Sleep onset delays slightly. Recovery becomes less efficient. Over months these shifts gradually erode margin.

An example clarifies this contrast. An individual consumes dinner at nine in the evening due to work schedule, followed by screen exposure and continued cognitive engagement. Sleep begins after midnight with minor fragmentation. Over time morning alertness decreases. Training output declines subtly. The feeding window itself is not harmful, but its alignment with circadian rhythm and workload compresses recovery.

In another case, early cessation of eating combined with late-night professional demands produces repeated bedtime hunger. The individual awakens during the night and struggles to return to sleep. The pattern repeats across weeks. Energy during the day feels adequate, yet adaptation stalls. The drift is not dramatic, but it is cumulative.

Sleep disruption narrows recovery margin because sleep is the primary period of repair and consolidation. When sleep becomes persistently fragmented or shortened, recovery kinetics slow. The system remains functional but less elastic.

Circadian misalignment under fasting does not represent a flaw in the timing structure itself. It reflects interaction between feeding schedule, workload, and biological rhythm. When alignment is preserved, fasting can coexist with stable sleep. When misalignment persists, small nightly disturbances accumulate into gradual stability erosion.

Circadian rhythm does more than regulate sleep onset. It organizes metabolic readiness across the day. Insulin sensitivity, digestive efficiency, cognitive alertness, and physical performance follow predictable arcs. When feeding timing repeatedly conflicts with these arcs, internal signals fragment. The system receives competing cues about when to mobilize and when to repair.

Fragmentation rarely appears dramatic at first. An individual may fall asleep each night yet wake slightly less restored. Morning readiness declines marginally. Evening alertness feels wired rather than calm. These shifts are subtle enough to normalize. Over months, however, the cost accumulates. Recovery no longer fully compensates for daily demand.

Circadian coherence also stabilizes appetite rhythm. When meals occur predictably during daylight hours and taper before biological night, hunger signals cluster appropriately. When meals extend late or fluctuate widely, hunger and satiety cues become less synchronized with sleep timing. This desynchronization can increase nighttime wakefulness or trigger early morning interruption.

The interaction between fasting and sleep is bidirectional. Compressed sleep can intensify hunger signaling the following day, which may alter feeding behavior within the window. Altered feeding then further shifts rhythm. Small deviations compound.

Consider a scenario of moderate misalignment. An individual adopts a feeding window that ends at 8 p.m., yet work extends until 10 p.m. Under moderate stress, the pattern remains tolerable. Under heightened stress, sleep onset delays and nighttime awakenings increase. The feeding structure is unchanged; the workload interaction reveals the instability.

Over time, minor nightly disruptions reduce total sleep by small increments. Thirty minutes lost each night accumulates into hours per week. Those hours represent recovery opportunity. As recovery compresses, performance and hormonal stability narrow in parallel. The erosion is incremental rather than catastrophic.

Circadian drift therefore acts as a slow amplifier of other stressors. What begins as a minor timing mismatch can become structural recovery compression when combined with high workload or marginal availability. The system loses coherence not because fasting is inherently destabilizing, but because feeding timing repeatedly conflicts with biological rhythm and environmental demand.

When energy availability narrows under stable conditions, the body often responds with proportional scaling. Output trims, metabolic rate calibrates, and signaling modulates coherently. The pattern remains orderly. When chronic sleep disruption and circadian misalignment enter the equation, the response becomes less orderly. Instead of smooth downregulation, volatility emerges.

Sleep functions as a regulatory stabilizer. During consolidated sleep, hormonal rhythms recalibrate. Cortisol declines, growth and repair signals rise, and appetite hormones reset. When sleep becomes fragmented or persistently shortened, this recalibration blurs. Rhythms that normally oscillate predictably begin to show noise.

Cortisol provides a clear illustration. Under stable alignment, cortisol peaks in the morning and tapers through the day. With chronic late-night eating combined with sustained stress, the evening decline may flatten. Cortisol remains modestly elevated at bedtime. Sleep becomes lighter or more fragmented. Morning peaks may feel exaggerated or muted. The rhythm is not absent; it is distorted.

Imagine an individual who routinely eats late due to work demands and continues cognitively demanding tasks into the night. Cortisol, elevated by workload, overlaps with digestion and screen exposure. The body attempts to transition toward sleep while stress signaling persists. Over weeks, the evening trough becomes less distinct. Morning wakefulness feels less crisp. The rhythm has lost clarity.

Appetite hormones respond similarly. Under coherent feeding windows and stable sleep, hunger anticipates predictable meals. Under inconsistent timing and fragmented sleep, hunger cues become less reliable. Some evenings bring intense hunger despite recent intake. Other days hunger is unexpectedly muted. The predictability that supports stable intake dissolves into oscillation.

An individual with inconsistent feeding windows may experience erratic hunger signaling. One day appetite peaks sharply at midday; the next it shifts toward late evening. Sleep disruption amplifies this variability. Leptin, ghrelin, and related signals rely on sleep for calibration. When sleep compresses, appetite often becomes louder or less synchronized with the feeding schedule.

Insulin sensitivity can fluctuate under similar conditions. Circadian misalignment and sleep restriction reduce glucose tolerance transiently. Meals consumed late at night may produce larger postprandial excursions than identical meals eaten earlier in the day. These shifts are not permanent impairments; they reflect context-dependent fluctuations in rhythmic alignment.

Reproductive signaling may also become more variable. Under coherent downregulation, cycles adjust proportionally and predictably. Under misalignment and sleep disruption, variability may increase. Cycle length may fluctuate without clear pattern as the system attempts to integrate competing signals of stress, feeding timing, and energy availability.

Increased sympathetic tone often accompanies chronic misalignment. When workload remains high and feeding windows compress recovery opportunity, the nervous system sustains mild vigilance. Restorative parasympathetic phases shorten. Mood may become more variable.

Emotional resilience narrows under minor stressors. These changes are subtle but perceptible.

The distinction between proportional scaling and instability lies in signal coherence. Proportional scaling produces orderly reduction in amplitude while preserving rhythm. Instability produces irregular oscillation and amplified noise. In one case signals are quieter but predictable. In the other they fluctuate unpredictably.

Sleep loss amplifies volatility because it removes nightly recalibration. Without consolidated sleep, hormonal rhythms lack a consistent reset point. Cortisol may spike at atypical times. Appetite may surge unexpectedly. Insulin sensitivity may vary day to day. The system becomes reactive rather than steady.

High workload layered onto fasting intensifies this volatility. Stress signaling remains elevated into evening hours. Feeding windows that end early may leave late-night hunger unresolved. Alternatively, feeding windows that extend late may collide with natural circadian decline. In both scenarios, integration of signals becomes noisy.

Mood variability often accompanies this state. An individual may feel energized and focused during fasting hours yet irritable by evening. Another may feel stable for several days and then experience abrupt dips in motivation. These fluctuations reflect cumulative signal distortion rather than isolated mood events.

One contrast clarifies the difference. In a state of stable downregulation under coherent marginal availability, performance plateaus while appetite remains predictable and mood steady. In a state of instability under chronic misalignment, appetite and mood oscillate unpredictably even if overall availability is similar. The difference lies in rhythm coherence.

Instability often precedes overt compression. Before performance ceiling narrows visibly, signal noise may increase. Hunger becomes less predictable. Sleep feels less restorative. Mood fluctuates more readily. These are early markers of misalignment rather than structural collapse.

Chronic misalignment therefore produces volatility rather than clean scaling. The body continues interpreting environmental signals, but without rhythmic coherence that interpretation fluctuates. Hormonal patterns amplify under load rather than modulate smoothly.

Signal instability often appears first as inconsistency rather than intensity. One week appetite feels exaggerated; the next it feels suppressed. One evening stress feels manageable; another it feels amplified without obvious cause. The variability itself becomes the marker. The system oscillates rather than settles.

When sleep becomes chronically fragmented, hormonal amplitude may increase while precision declines. Cortisol peaks may occur at less predictable times. Hunger may emerge independent of meal timing. Without rhythmic anchoring, physiology develops a subtle jitter. This jitter can feel like heightened sensitivity to everyday events.

Erratic hunger under inconsistent windows provides a practical example. An individual may follow a fasting structure during the workweek but allow irregular timing on weekends. Sleep shifts slightly later. Appetite cues drift. By Monday, hunger timing no longer aligns cleanly with the feeding window. The body attempts to recalibrate, but repeated minor shifts prevent stable entrainment. Oscillation replaces steady rhythm.

Late-night cognitive engagement combined with compressed feeding can also distort the normal tapering of activation. An individual may feel wired late into the evening and unusually sluggish mid-morning. These reversals are not pathological; they reflect competing cues struggling for dominance.

Volatility differs from clean downregulation in its unpredictability. Under proportional scaling the system becomes quieter but stable. Under instability signals may feel louder yet inconsistent. Appetite surges are followed by muted days. Motivation spikes give way to disproportionate dips. The organism is not failing to regulate; it is regulating against conflicting inputs.

Over time this signaling noise increases overall strain. Because cues are less predictable, behavioral consistency becomes harder to maintain. Feeding timing may shift in response to hunger volatility, which further destabilizes rhythm. Mood variability can alter sleep timing, amplifying endocrine fluctuation. Small oscillations compound.

High workload magnifies these effects because stress signaling overlaps with feeding and sleep timing. The nervous system remains activated when it should be tapering. Without adequate recovery anchoring the cycle, endocrine rhythms become more reactive and less synchronized.

The distinction is subtle but important. Stable marginal availability produces coherent scaling. Chronic misalignment produces incoherent oscillation. One narrows capacity quietly. The other injects noise into regulation, making stability harder to preserve.

Hormonal instability under chronic misalignment therefore reflects signaling noise and volatility arising from disrupted rhythmic integration rather than inherent endocrine dysfunction.

Structure can stabilize behavior. Predictable timing reduces decision load and organizes intake within defined boundaries. When integrated proportionally, this structure supports coherence across metabolic and psychological domains. Under sustained instability, however, structure can gradually harden into rigidity.

The distinction between structured and rigid is subtle but consequential. Structured timing allows adjustment when demands change. It tolerates deviation without destabilizing identity or producing disproportionate distress. Rigid timing resists adjustment. Deviation feels threatening. The structure shifts from scaffold to enforcement.

Plateau often becomes the inflection point. When performance stalls or body composition remains unchanged despite adherence, interpretation of that plateau determines the next trajectory. If plateau is viewed as completion of adaptation, structure may remain stable. If plateau is interpreted as insufficient effort, tightening often follows.

Incremental window compression frequently unfolds quietly. A ten-hour feeding window becomes eight. Eight becomes six. The initial reduction feels manageable and even clarifying. Hunger concentrates but remains tolerable. Results may appear to accelerate briefly due to novelty effects or early water shifts. When progress slows again, another reduction may follow.

Five hours replaces six. Eventually the structure narrows to a point where recovery margin compresses.

An individual who began with a moderate twelve-hour eating span might gradually compress intake to a four-hour window across several months. Each shift feels logical in the moment, framed as refinement rather than intensification. Yet each compression reduces opportunity for restoration, social flexibility, and contextual adaptation.

Plateau interpreted as insufficient discipline intensifies this pattern. Rather than examining broader proportional variables, the conclusion forms that greater control will solve stagnation. The sense of agency increases with tightening. Control feels productive. Hunger tolerance becomes proof of commitment. The structure appears to offer a clear lever to pull.

Under instability—whether physiological volatility from misalignment or subtle performance compression—control seeking often amplifies. The mind searches for adjustable variables. Timing is visible and easily modified. Compressing the window provides immediate action. The psychological relief of doing something can mask the structural consequences.

Feedback loops develop between instability and rigidity. Sleep fragmentation or appetite volatility creates discomfort. The response becomes further tightening. The additional tightening increases physiological strain. Strain amplifies instability. The cycle repeats. Each step appears rational in isolation. Cumulatively, the loop narrows flexibility.

Psychological load increases even if intake remains similar. Rigid timing requires vigilance. Social events become obstacles. Meals outside predetermined windows create internal tension. The feeding structure gradually becomes the central organizing principle.

An example illustrates this shift. An individual who once adjusted meal timing flexibly around social commitments begins declining invitations because they fall outside the eating window. The choice feels protective of progress. Over time social engagement decreases. The structure remains intact, yet adaptability shrinks.

Rigidity reduces resilience because resilience depends on tolerance for variability. When structure cannot accommodate minor perturbations, small deviations produce disproportionate stress. A delayed meal triggers anxiety. An unexpected late meeting creates internal conflict. The metabolic contour may remain similar, but psychological strain increases.

Flexible structure operates differently. When timing supports rhythm without dominating identity, modest adjustments remain possible. If workload rises temporarily or social context shifts, the window adapts slightly without loss of coherence. Hunger signals become information rather than threat. The structure serves the system instead of constraining it.

Escalation cycles often arise from the illusion that discipline resolves physiological compression. When performance narrows or appetite becomes unpredictable, intensifying restriction appears to restore control. In practice, further compression may reduce recovery margin and amplify instability.

The incremental nature of escalation obscures its impact. Each reduction feels small. The cumulative narrowing can meaningfully constrain adaptability. Recovery windows shorten. Social flexibility declines. Psychological preoccupation increases. Yet because the structure itself remains consistent, the pattern can appear stable.

Under stress, rigid structures tend to tighten further. Instead of expanding to absorb variability, they contract. Internal pressure increases. Elasticity declines.

Contrast this with a flexible structure under similar stress. When workload rises temporarily, feeding timing may shift slightly to preserve recovery. Identity remains intact because it is not defined exclusively by the window. Structure adapts to context. Stability persists.

Psychological rigidity and escalation cycles are not inherent to fasting. They emerge when structure is treated as the primary solution to plateau or instability. When identity attaches tightly to timing boundaries, flexibility narrows. Instability then feeds further tightening.

When instability appears—whether as plateau, mood variability, appetite unpredictability, or subtle performance compression—the impulse to tighten structure often follows. Tightening feels corrective. It introduces clarity where uncertainty exists. Yet when escalation occurs in the presence of compromised recovery or misalignment, the result is not refinement but amplification.

Escalation functions as compensatory behavior. A narrower feeding window, a longer fasting interval, or more rigid adherence appears to restore order. In the short term it can create a sense of control. Hunger may initially sharpen and then mute. Daily structure feels decisive. However, when sleep is fragmented or workload remains elevated, additional compression reduces recovery margin further.

Compressed windows layered onto poor sleep create cumulative strain. If late nights already shorten restoration time, further restricting feeding duration concentrates intake into a narrower span and extends fasting into hours of heightened stress. The sympathetic nervous system, already activated by insufficient sleep, encounters prolonged energy gaps. The result is not immediate collapse but elevated baseline tension.

Low availability combined with high stress load increases physiological vigilance. Cortisol rhythm may remain less distinct. Appetite signals can grow louder or more erratic. Hunger that once followed predictable timing begins to spike unexpectedly. Under these conditions escalating discipline does not calm the system; it often intensifies oscillation.

Consider an individual under occupational strain who compresses a previously moderate feeding window from eight hours to five. Sleep has already shortened due to workload. Training volume remains high. For several days the change feels empowering. By the third or fourth week recovery lag extends. Minor perturbations—an extra meeting or a delayed meal—produce disproportionate fatigue. Hunger becomes sharper late in the evening and begins to intrude on sleep. The attempt to regain control through tightening amplifies physiological strain.

Performance compression can intensify this loop. When output declines, tightening appears logical. A plateau in strength or endurance may be interpreted as insufficient precision. The feeding window narrows further while training remains demanding. Reduced adaptive range under stress diminishes responsiveness to stimulus. Output stagnates or declines further. The perceived solution—more restriction—feeds the condition it attempts to correct.

Appetite volatility worsens under escalating restriction when recovery remains compromised. Hunger signals amplified by sleep loss and stress collide with tighter timing boundaries. The result can be alternating phases of strict adherence and concentrated intake within the window. The individual experiences this as inconsistency, yet the pattern reflects amplified signaling rather than lack of resolve.

The distinction between stable tightening and destabilizing tightening lies in context. Under stable sleep, moderate workload, and adequate availability, modest compression may integrate without narrowing flexibility. Under stacked stress and reduced recovery, further tightening compounds strain. Identical structural changes produce different physiological outcomes depending on alignment.

Another example illustrates this divergence. Two individuals reduce feeding duration from ten hours to seven. One maintains consistent sleep and moderate training. Recovery remains intact. Appetite stabilizes after brief adjustment. The other increases training intensity while sleep remains compressed. Hunger becomes erratic. Recovery slows. Mood fluctuates. The same structural change interacts with load differently in each case.

Escalation cycles often develop gradually. Initial tightening produces temporary reinforcement. Early effects—perhaps minor weight fluctuation or sharper hunger cues—feel meaningful. When these effects normalize, further tightening follows. Each cycle reduces recovery margin incrementally. Because the changes are small, the narrowing often goes unnoticed.

Physiological strain under escalation is cumulative. Sympathetic tone may remain elevated longer into the evening. Sleep onset may delay slightly. Minor nightly disruptions accumulate. Recovery kinetics lengthen subtly. Adaptive range narrows. The system becomes less tolerant of variability.

Flexibility functions as protective architecture. When structure allows modest adjustment in response to stress or workload spikes, recovery can be preserved. When escalation replaces adjustment, elasticity diminishes. Behavioral tightening amplifies physiological instability, which then reinforces behavioral tightening.

Appetite volatility offers a clear marker of this amplification. Under escalating restriction layered onto stress, hunger may oscillate sharply—muted during the day and intense at night. Episodes of concentrated intake within the window become more likely. The volatility may be interpreted as a need for further discipline, perpetuating the loop.

Escalation does not inherently produce harm. It becomes destabilizing when it substitutes for restoration. Without realignment of sleep, workload, or availability, tightening structure narrows the bandwidth required for stability.

Instability rarely begins with collapse. It begins with drift. The architecture of daily rhythm, appetite, performance, and mood shifts subtly before overt compression appears. Because these shifts are incremental, they are easily absorbed into routine and interpreted as normal variation.

Sleep drift often appears first. Bedtime extends slightly later. Sleep onset becomes less immediate. Night awakenings increase modestly. Morning alertness feels fractionally muted. None of these changes alone signal failure. They resemble ordinary fluctuation. When they repeat across weeks, however, they reflect cumulative misalignment rather than isolated disturbance.

An individual who once fell asleep within minutes may begin scrolling longer before rest. The final meal occurs closer to bedtime as schedules compress. Work extends further into the evening. Sleep still occurs, but its depth changes subtly. Morning energy declines slightly. Training feels marginally heavier. The drift is gradual enough to feel ordinary.

Appetite volatility may follow. Hunger signals lose predictability. Some days begin with muted appetite and end with intense evening hunger. Other days reverse the pattern. The feeding window remains intact, yet internal cues feel noisier. What was once steady becomes erratic. Because timing remains consistent, the instability may be attributed to stress or distraction rather than structural strain.

Performance stagnation under consistent stimulus provides another early indicator. Workload remains constant. Training volume does not increase. Yet progress halts. Effort rises slightly to maintain the same output. The plateau is interpreted as completion of adaptation or as a need for further tightening. Rarely is it recognized as a signal of compressed margin.

Mood variability may narrow tolerance as well. Minor frustrations evoke stronger responses. Emotional resilience thins. The system remains functional but less elastic. Recovery from stress requires more time. These shifts accumulate quietly rather than appearing as dramatic changes.

Loss of variability tolerance reflects deeper structural narrowing. Occasional late meals or schedule shifts that were once absorbed easily now produce disproportionate disruption. Social events feel harder to integrate. Timing becomes less flexible. Internal tension rises around deviations that were previously manageable.

Increasing preoccupation with timing often accompanies this narrowing. The feeding window occupies more cognitive bandwidth. Meals are evaluated more strictly. Minor deviations feel significant. The structure that once supported rhythm begins to dominate attention.

Reduced recovery elasticity emerges in small ways. Minor illnesses linger longer. Muscle soreness resolves more slowly. Cognitive clarity returns later in the day. These changes rarely provoke alarm. They blend gradually into routine.

Plateau accompanied by rising effort illustrates the pattern clearly. An individual increases training intensity slightly while maintaining compressed feeding. Output does not improve. Effort increases. Fatigue accumulates modestly. The response may be further tightening of structure, even though the underlying issue lies in compressed margin rather than insufficient discipline.

Recognition of sleep drift can mark the beginning of reversal. An individual notices that bedtime has shifted progressively later and morning alertness has dulled. Instead of intensifying structure, feeding timing adjusts slightly to better align with workload and rest. Within weeks sleep onset improves. Morning energy stabilizes. The relief feels disproportionate to the small adjustment, revealing how narrow the margin had become.

Appetite becoming noisier offers another example. Evening hunger spikes under compressed feeding combined with late stress. A modest widening of structure—or slightly greater restoration relative to workload—reduces volatility. Hunger becomes predictable again. The change feels like quiet stabilization rather than dramatic improvement.

Realignment often begins with restoration dominance across cycles. When recovery opportunity increases and feeding timing aligns more closely with circadian rhythm, oscillations smooth. Mood steadies. Performance responds gradually. The return of elasticity usually precedes visible performance gains.

One individual experiencing plateau and rising effort broadens the feeding window modestly while moderating workload temporarily. Within weeks recovery lag shortens. Training output resumes upward trajectory. The change feels like relief rather than concession. Structure remains present, but it regains flexibility.

Contrast this with escalation. Under escalation tightening continues despite drift. Sleep worsens. Appetite volatility intensifies. Plateau persists. Effort increases further. Under realignment margin widens subtly. Recovery improves. Variability tolerance returns. The system once again absorbs disturbance without disproportionate strain.

Flexibility signals resilience. The ability to widen or shift structure without distress reflects preserved adaptive capacity. Realignment does not require abandoning fasting. It requires restoring coherence between feeding timing, workload, and recovery.

Early signals appear before collapse because the system prioritizes preservation. Downward drift is gradual. Reversal is equally gradual. Relief often accompanies realignment because internal tension decreases. The architecture regains proportion. Relief is the first sign that the system is re-cohering.

Training, Workload, and Energy Demand

Fasting does not operate in isolation. It intersects with energy demand, and energy demand is not constant across individuals or across seasons of life. The same feeding window can exist inside radically different energetic environments. Without context, timing appears uniform. Within context, its meaning changes.

Energy demand includes more than visible exertion. It encompasses physical labor, structured training, cognitive intensity, emotional strain, and environmental exposure. Some forms are obvious. Others are subtle but metabolically significant.

A construction worker engaged in manual labor experiences continuous muscular demand across the workday. Lifting, carrying, climbing, and stabilizing generate steady energy flux. Even when movements are not maximal, they are sustained. In this context, fasting compresses intake into fewer hours while demand persists across many. The relationship between timing and restoration becomes critical because output is not intermittent; it is continuous.

Contrast this with a desk professional. Hours may pass with minimal movement. Energy expenditure is lower, even if stress is present. A compressed feeding window in this environment may feel seamless because output does not outpace intake opportunity in the same way. Hunger may be manageable. Recovery may not feel constrained. Identical timing, different demand.

Cognitive load complicates the picture further. High-level decision-making, sustained attention, and emotional regulation require metabolic resources even when physical movement is limited. A trial attorney preparing arguments for extended periods, a surgeon navigating complex procedures, or a financial analyst managing volatile markets may experience substantial neural demand. Brain glucose utilization increases under sustained cognitive work. Fasting in such contexts interacts with concentration, mood, and decision resilience differently than it does in lower cognitive-load environments.

A high-intensity athlete provides another lens. Structured training sessions generate concentrated demand. Outside training, recovery becomes the primary process. If feeding timing does not align with training schedule, mismatch emerges. A compressed feeding window that ends before late-afternoon training may leave limited restoration opportunity before sleep. Alternatively, early training combined with delayed intake may prolong a post-exertion shortfall. Demand magnitude interacts with intake timing in ways that alter tolerance.

Shift workers introduce another variable. A nurse working overnight encounters circadian inversion. Energy demand occurs when biological readiness is reduced. Feeding windows layered onto this schedule may intersect awkwardly with sleep. Fasting tolerance under such circumstances differs from that of a daytime worker with stable rhythm. The same eight-hour window may be restorative in one environment and destabilizing in another.

Total load exceeds visible exertion. An individual caring for young children while managing employment may carry constant low-level demand. Sleep fragmentation compounds this load. By contrast, someone with predictable hours and minimal external stress may maintain stable demand even with moderate physical activity. Timing that integrates smoothly in one context may compress margin in another.

Demand timing matters as much as magnitude. A manual laborer whose heaviest workload occurs mid-morning may tolerate delayed intake differently than one whose workload peaks late afternoon. An athlete training early morning may integrate feeding differently than one training in the evening. The alignment between output peaks and intake windows shapes stability.

Energy availability is relational. It cannot be evaluated solely by total intake; it must be considered relative to expenditure pattern and timing. A fasting window that coincides with low-demand hours may feel sustainable. The same window imposed during peak demand may narrow margin.

Workload escalation changes fasting tolerance. An individual may integrate a six-hour window comfortably during a sedentary period. When workload increases—through training, occupational change, or life stress—the same window may begin to strain recovery. No visible change in timing occurs, yet context shifts its interpretation.

Consider two individuals adopting identical eight-hour feeding windows. One works in construction, lifting and moving materials from dawn until mid-afternoon. Intake occurs late afternoon and evening. The other works at a computer with moderate activity. For the laborer, extended morning demand without intake may increase fatigue and amplify evening hunger. For the desk worker, morning fasting may feel neutral. The window is identical; the environment is not.

Similarly, a high-intensity athlete compressing intake into evening hours while training twice daily may encounter slower recovery kinetics than during a lower-volume phase. When training volume decreases in the off-season, the same timing structure may integrate without strain. The variable is not discipline; it is demand.

A shift worker who rotates schedules may find fasting manageable during day shifts but destabilizing during night rotations. Appetite rhythms, sleep opportunity, and energy demand shift simultaneously. Identical structure interacts differently with altered context.

Matched timing aligns intake opportunity with output peaks and recovery windows. Mismatched timing concentrates intake away from demand or compresses restoration into already narrow intervals. The difference may be subtle at first but accumulates across weeks.

Continuous muscular work illustrates this clearly. A laborer lifting and moving material from early morning onward generates steady substrate turnover. If intake does not occur until late afternoon, mobilization sustains output for hours. Over days this may feel manageable. Over weeks, recovery quality becomes the determinant. If restoration later in the day does not fully compensate for extended morning demand, compression unfolds quietly.

Cognitive demand presents a different but related pattern. Sustained decision-making, emotional regulation, and complex reasoning require stable energy availability. When prolonged fasting overlaps peak cognitive workload, clarity may initially feel sharp due to catecholamine elevation. Over time, however, oscillation may increase. Late-day fatigue may intensify. Hunger may intrude into focus. The mismatch lies not in total intake but in temporal alignment.

Seasonal workload shifts amplify this dynamic. An athlete during the off-season may tolerate extended fasting windows because training intensity and volume are lower. Entering a competitive phase increases both the magnitude and timing sensitivity of demand. A previously neutral feeding structure may begin to constrain recovery. The structure did not change; the environment did.

Life-phase transitions create similar shifts. A new parent experiencing fragmented sleep may find a formerly stable window increasingly difficult to integrate. A promotion that increases decision density changes cognitive expenditure. A move from desk work to more active labor alters muscular demand. In each case, identical timing interacts with altered context.

Demand clustering also matters. High-intensity efforts create concentrated energy flux even if total daily expenditure is moderate. A desk professional who performs a single intense training session after work may encounter different restoration dynamics than a person performing moderate physical activity distributed throughout the day. The timing of that session relative to the intake window shapes recovery trajectory.

Tolerance can be context-dependent without being fragile. A feeding window that functions smoothly during stable workload may require adjustment during escalation. Recognizing this variability reflects adaptive intelligence rather than inconsistency. The system responds to relational proportion, not to ideological adherence.

Baseline functioning and peak output are not the same condition. Baseline reflects the capacity to complete routine tasks, sustain moderate movement, and maintain stable cognition. Peak output requires mobilization beyond baseline. It demands rapid substrate flux, neuromuscular precision, and coordinated signaling. The difference often becomes visible only under strain.

High-intensity output differs fundamentally from steady, lower-intensity demand. Sprinting, heavy lifting, or explosive movement relies heavily on rapid glycolytic flux and stored glycogen. Steady endurance efforts draw more broadly from mixed substrates and can be sustained under wider conditions. When fuel timing aligns with the nature of demand, the system operates smoothly. When misaligned, ceiling narrows before baseline fails.

Consider early-morning high-intensity training performed in a fasted state. Upon waking, catecholamines are naturally elevated. Alertness is high. Mobilization pathways are primed. The session may feel sharp and efficient. For a single bout, output can be strong. Yet repeated high-intensity sessions without prior fuel may increase recovery cost. Glycogen depletion accumulates. Restoration windows shorten if intake remains delayed. Performance may appear stable at first, then plateau subtly.

In contrast, a fed state before high-intensity output can feel heavier at onset. Insulin has risen. Digestive processes are active. Subjective lightness may be reduced. Yet substrate availability supports rapid energy production. Recovery kinetics may improve. The session may not feel sharper, but cumulative adaptation may differ.

Neither state is inherently superior. Their interaction with workload volume, frequency, and recovery capacity determines outcome. When fasted high-intensity sessions occur occasionally within ample restoration context, adaptation can proceed without visible compression. When such sessions repeat under heavy workload, recovery margin narrows.

Cognitive performance windows reflect similar dynamics. An individual working intensely on analytical tasks during a morning fast may experience heightened focus due to elevated catecholamines. Alertness can feel pronounced. Distraction decreases. Yet sustained cognitive throughput across many hours may decline if energy availability remains limited relative to demand. Perceived sharpness at onset does not always translate to sustained output.

An afternoon cognitive peak under fasting can illustrate this nuance. For several hours, concentration feels clean and uninterrupted. As tasks extend, mental fatigue accumulates more rapidly than on days when intake preceded peak work. The difference is subtle but cumulative. Baseline cognition remains intact; the ceiling narrows slightly.

The contrast between endurance and sprinting clarifies fuel-timing interaction. A steady-state run performed fasted may feel stable, drawing on mixed substrates. The same individual attempting maximal sprint intervals under identical conditions may experience reduced peak power or slower recovery between efforts. Misalignment can remain invisible at moderate intensity and become obvious only at maximal demand.

Repeated fasted high-intensity training layered onto heavy occupational workload compounds this effect. A construction worker who trains intensely before dawn and then performs manual labor all day operates under sustained demand. Initially, the routine feels disciplined and efficient. Over weeks, subtle compression appears. Recovery between sessions slows. Evening fatigue intensifies. Appetite volatility increases. The mismatch between fuel timing and cumulative demand narrows the adaptive envelope.

High-intensity output amplifies these interactions because it relies on rapid substrate availability. Anaerobic bursts deplete localized stores quickly. Without timely restoration, repeated efforts draw from shrinking reserve. Steady demand tolerates wider timing variation, yet chronic misalignment can still reduce maximal capacity before affecting routine performance.

Fuel timing influences how adaptive signals are interpreted. When substrate availability aligns with demand peaks, adaptation tends toward expansion. When misaligned persistently, adaptation shifts toward conservation. The difference may be small in single sessions but significant across cycles.

Acute performance and cumulative adaptation do not always move together. A session performed fasted may feel efficient—even powerful—due to elevated sympathetic tone. Heart rate rises readily. Mobilization feels immediate. Output in short bursts may appear unaffected. Yet adaptation depends not only on the session but on how the system interprets the session afterward.

When high-intensity work repeatedly occurs in a low-availability state, the adaptive signal can shift. Instead of registering the effort as an expansion stimulus supported by adequate restoration, the system may interpret it as strain requiring cautious allocation. Recovery prioritizes preservation rather than amplification. Gains slow not because effort was insufficient, but because context signaled constraint.

Neural fatigue adds another dimension. High cognitive output or technical training requires precise neural signaling. Even when muscular recovery appears adequate, central fatigue can accumulate if substrate timing consistently trails peak cognitive demand. Focus becomes more effortful. Reaction speed diminishes slightly. These shifts may be too small to detect in routine tasks but appear under competitive or high-stakes conditions.

Recovery cost is often asymmetric. The energetic cost of high-intensity output is immediate and concentrated. The restoration cost is distributed and delayed. When intake timing consistently postpones replenishment after peak demand, lag compounds. Each session may seem manageable, yet the cumulative recovery shortfall accumulates invisibly.

Repeated mismatch under dense workload accelerates this process. An individual balancing demanding occupational output with structured training may tolerate occasional fasted high-intensity work. When such sessions become routine under already elevated stress, cumulative load increases total system strain. Sleep quality may decline subtly. Appetite volatility may increase. Performance plateau may precede obvious fatigue.

Ceiling erosion often appears first in efforts requiring maximal coordination or repeatability. Sprint intervals lose slight power. Heavy lifts feel less explosive. Complex cognitive tasks require more deliberate pacing. Baseline remains intact. Narrowing becomes detectable only at the edges of capacity.

By contrast, when fuel timing aligns more consistently with demand peaks, adaptive signals are clearer. High-intensity output is followed by proportionate restoration. Neural and muscular recovery synchronize more efficiently. Performance variability decreases under repeated stress.

The distinction is not binary but relational. A fasted morning interval may integrate well when overall load is moderate and recovery ample. The same interval may contribute to compression when layered onto high-density workload without adjustment.

Alignment therefore shapes not just immediate output but the meaning the body assigns to that output. When strain is paired with restoration, expansion becomes more likely. When strain is layered onto prolonged low availability, conservation may predominate.

Fuel timing shapes performance not through any moral superiority of fed or fasted states, but through alignment between substrate availability and demand peaks. When alignment is preserved, adaptive response integrates efficiently. When misalignment persists under high demand, ceiling narrows quietly.

Fuel timing operates as a performance-alignment variable whose impact depends on contextual demand and recovery integration rather than as a categorical choice between fed and fasted states.

Energy demand expresses itself differently across occupations. Some work is visibly physical. Some is cognitively dense. Some is emotionally absorbing. Each produces a pattern of turnover that interacts with feeding structure in distinct ways.

Continuous muscular flux characterizes manual labor. A construction worker lifting lumber, climbing scaffolding, stabilizing loads, and walking uneven terrain experiences sustained contraction across large muscle groups. Movements are not necessarily maximal, but they are repeated across hours. Energy turnover is steady. Glycogen is drawn upon, replenished, and drawn again. Even in moments of pause, the body remains engaged.

In this environment, fasting tolerance reflects more than discipline. It reflects alignment between continuous demand and restoration windows. If intake is compressed into a narrow span after long hours of labor, recovery must compete with accumulated fatigue and sleep onset. Over time, small mismatches between demand timing and feeding timing may narrow margin.

A factory worker on a long shift encounters similar flux. Repetitive lifting, standing, or machine operation produces continuous low-to-moderate muscular output. Expenditure is not dramatic, yet it accumulates across the day. Unlike episodic training, which ends and allows discrete recovery, occupational demand persists.

Sedentary work appears different. A software engineer may sit for most of the day. Visible movement is limited. Energy expenditure is lower than manual labor. Yet sedentary does not mean demand-free.

Cognitive strain consumes metabolic resources in subtler ways. Sustained attention, problem-solving, and rapid decision-making elevate neural glucose utilization. Stress associated with deadlines or complex tasks activates sympathetic pathways. Although total caloric expenditure remains modest compared to manual labor, demand pattern can still compress margin when layered onto restricted intake and limited sleep.

An office worker under cognitive strain may report fatigue by late afternoon despite minimal movement. The fatigue differs from muscular exhaustion, yet it reflects continuous neural activation. When fasting windows extend through peak cognitive hours, the experience may initially feel sharp due to catecholamine elevation. Over time, sustained mismatch between cognitive load and intake timing can reduce resilience to stressors.

Emotional labor adds another dimension. A nurse working a hospital floor engages in physical tasks—walking, lifting, adjusting patients—while simultaneously regulating emotion, responding to crises, and maintaining composure. Emotional regulation carries metabolic cost. It activates stress pathways. Recovery between interactions may be minimal during long shifts.

A therapist or customer service professional may remain seated yet expend significant psychological energy. Holding attention, moderating tone, and absorbing client stress require sustained neural engagement. This invisible expenditure contributes to cumulative demand.

Continuous low-level fatigue differs from episodic spikes. A high-intensity training session produces a clear demand peak followed by defined recovery. Continuous occupational output produces steady drain without obvious climax. The body adapts by smoothing energy allocation across hours. Fasting in this context shifts restoration opportunity relative to that drain.

A construction worker who eats only late evening after a full day of labor may initially tolerate the schedule. Over weeks, subtle signs appear: slower evening recovery, increased appetite volatility, slightly delayed sleep onset. The mismatch lies not in the window alone but in the relationship between continuous demand and delayed restoration.

An office worker may tolerate a similar window without overt compression because mechanical output is lower. However, under intense project deadlines, cognitive demand escalates. Sleep shortens. Fasting tolerance shifts. The same window that felt neutral during moderate workload now interacts with compressed recovery.

A nurse on rotating shifts encounters both physical and circadian strain. Continuous movement combines with night rotations. Feeding windows layered onto this schedule may amplify fatigue if restoration aligns poorly with shift timing. Work structure, not visible intensity alone, shapes tolerance.

The sedentary illusion arises when low visible movement is equated with low demand. Desk work can conceal substantial cognitive and emotional load. Fatigue at day's end may be attributed to inactivity, yet it often reflects sustained neural engagement. Fasting under these conditions may feel sustainable until stress accumulates.

Perceived fatigue does not always mirror energetic reality. A manual laborer may feel physically tired yet metabolically aligned if feeding matches demand. An office worker may feel less physically fatigued yet metabolically strained if cognitive load coincides with prolonged fasting and sleep compression.

Recovery timing interacts with occupational structure. Jobs with predictable breaks allow intermittent restoration. Continuous shifts without breaks compress recovery into evening hours. When feeding windows also concentrate intake late, restoration must share space with sleep preparation.

Continuous output narrows margin faster than episodic spikes because it offers fewer distinct recovery phases. Sedentary contexts may tolerate compression differently, but hidden fatigue can still accumulate under cognitive and emotional strain.

Continuous demand changes the recovery equation because it lacks sharp boundaries. A structured training session ends. Muscular activation declines. Recovery signaling begins clearly. Occupational labor rarely ends in such discrete fashion. Movement tapers gradually. Neural engagement lingers. Stress signaling fades slowly rather than abruptly. The body can enter evening hours already partially depleted without a clear transition point.

This blurring of demand and recovery phases increases the importance of timing alignment. When restoration is delayed after a day of continuous flux, the gap between expenditure and replenishment widens subtly. Even if total intake later matches expenditure, the prolonged interval between demand and restoration can influence sleep depth and recovery kinetics.

Adaptive masking often occurs in sedentary contexts. Because visible exertion is low, fasting tolerance may appear robust. Energy feels stable. Hunger may be manageable. However, when stress density increases—tight deadlines, emotional strain, prolonged decision-making—margin may narrow without obvious physical signs. Compression becomes visible only when performance under pressure declines.

Continuous output narrows margin faster because it erodes micro-recovery opportunities. Small breaks in muscular labor or cognitive focus function as mini-restorative intervals. When work intensity or duration reduces these intervals, cumulative load rises. If feeding timing does not compensate proportionally, recovery becomes increasingly backloaded into limited evening hours.

Shift-based manual work adds another complexity. A nurse finishing a twelve-hour night shift may enter a feeding window at biological times not optimized for digestion or sleep. Even if intake is adequate, circadian misalignment alters how efficiently restoration integrates. Demand structure interacts with both timing and rhythm.

Emotional labor compounds this pattern. Sustained affect regulation activates stress pathways repeatedly across a shift. These activations may be brief but frequent. Repeated across hours, they resemble continuous low-level sympathetic tone. Fasting layered onto such a pattern may feel manageable at first yet reduce tolerance to additional stressors.

The difference between episodic and continuous demand becomes especially clear under escalation. Adding structured training to an already physically demanding occupation may compress margin more rapidly than expected. The body integrates total load, not just planned exercise.

Fasting tolerance is not static. It evolves alongside training cycles, occupational demands, sleep architecture, and age-related shifts in recovery. A structure that integrates smoothly during one season may compress margin during another, even when the structure itself is unchanged.

Early success often occurs during periods of relatively low demand. An athlete in the off-season, training moderately and sleeping consistently, may adopt a compressed feeding window without noticeable strain. Recovery remains intact. Performance feels stable. Appetite aligns predictably. The structure appears universally effective.

When competitive season arrives, training volume intensifies. Travel increases. Sleep fragments. Psychological load rises. The same feeding window that once felt neutral now overlaps peak demand and shortened recovery. Subtle compression appears: slower recovery between sessions, increased evening hunger, minor mood variability. The structure did not change; the environment did.

A similar shift can occur with career transitions. An individual who maintained stable fasting under predictable workload may receive a promotion. Responsibility increases. Meetings extend later. Cognitive load intensifies. Sleep onset shifts slightly. The feeding window remains intact, yet appetite becomes less predictable. Performance remains adequate but requires more effort. Over months, margin narrows quietly.

New parenthood illustrates a distinct pattern. Sleep fragmentation becomes routine. Night awakenings compress restoration. Emotional demand increases. Even if workload remains constant, cumulative sleep loss alters tolerance. A feeding structure that once aligned comfortably with daily rhythm may now collide with irregular sleep and unpredictable stress. Hunger timing shifts. Recovery feels incomplete. The structure is unchanged; the life phase is not.

Aging adds further modulation. Recovery kinetics lengthen gradually. Muscle repair slows modestly. Sleep becomes lighter. Hormonal rhythms shift subtly. A fasting pattern tolerated easily in early adulthood may compress margin in later years without visible change in intake or timing. The system's capacity for rapid oscillation narrows, requiring proportionate restoration to preserve elasticity.

Stress density accumulation functions similarly. Multiple small demands—work pressure, family obligations, travel—create a background load that may not be individually disruptive. Together, they compress recovery opportunity. Fasting tolerance under low stress may not predict tolerance under cumulative stress.

Workload escalation without intake or timing change often exposes mismatch. An athlete increasing training volume while maintaining identical feeding structure may initially feel disciplined. Over weeks, performance plateaus earlier. Recovery lag increases. Appetite volatility rises. The adaptive capacity that supported earlier integration now encounters narrower margin.

Identical structure compresses margin later because adaptive capacity changes. The body recalibrates to context. A feeding window is not evaluated in isolation but relative to demand, sleep, and stress environment. What once represented proportionate restriction may become marginal availability when demand increases.

Early success can mask later mismatch. When fasting integrates during a low-demand phase, it may appear universally compatible. This perception persists even as context shifts. Structural inertia develops: the assumption that what worked once must work indefinitely.

Structural integrity differs from structural inertia. Integrity reflects alignment between timing and context. Inertia reflects adherence despite context shift. The difference is not visible in the window itself but in the relationship between window and environment.

An athlete transitioning from off-season to peak season provides a clear contrast. In the off-season, moderate training aligns with compressed intake. In peak season, training intensifies. A flexible approach integrates additional restoration around peak sessions. A static approach preserves the original window rigidly. Over time, the static approach narrows recovery margin, while flexible integration preserves capacity.

New parent sleep fragmentation shows how life phases alter baseline capacity. Feeding timing that once supported stable appetite rhythm may now interact unpredictably with night awakenings. Flexibility absorbs this variability. Inertia resists adaptation.

Age-related recovery shift often unfolds gradually. An individual in midlife may notice slower post-training restoration despite identical intake and timing. The margin that once supported compression now requires proportionate expansion. Structural inertia may interpret this as failure of discipline rather than change in context.

Adaptive mismatch is not binary. It is gradual and contextual. Tolerance during one season does not guarantee tolerance during another. Adaptive capacity shifts with workload, sleep, age, and stress density.

Stress stacking intensifies this dynamic. Career advancement may coincide with relocation. Parenting demands may coincide with disrupted sleep and financial pressure. Aging may coincide with higher occupational responsibility. Each variable adds density. The cumulative effect reduces margin even if intake and timing remain constant.

The consequences of mismatch are often first visible at performance edges. An athlete notices reduced repeatability under peak load. A professional notices decision fatigue earlier in the day. A parent notices irritability under minor stressors. Baseline remains intact; elasticity diminishes.

Over time, repeated minor mismatches become pattern. The organism does not abruptly fail; it gradually reallocates. Recovery windows lengthen. Variability tolerance shrinks. Appetite rhythm becomes noisier. Sleep becomes lighter. None of these changes alone require alarm. Together, they signal contextual shift.

Flexibility does not require abandoning structure. It requires recognizing that structure exists within moving terrain. When terrain shifts and structure does not, compression results. When structure adapts proportionally, stability persists.

Adaptive mismatch emerges not from a defect in timing itself but from the natural evolution of workload, age, stress density, and life complexity. The variable is dynamic. The structure must integrate that dynamism to preserve margin.

Fasting structure does not exist in a vacuum. It lives inside workload patterns, sleep architecture, cognitive demand, emotional strain, and life-phase transitions. Across these shifting variables, stability is determined not by uniform adherence but by proportional alignment.

Proportion is relational. It is not defined by feeding-window length alone, nor by rigidity. It is defined by how intake timing interacts with energy demand and recovery opportunity across cycles. When alignment is preserved, margin remains intact. When alignment drifts, ceiling narrows first.

Early success often reflects favorable proportion. During a period of moderate workload and consistent sleep, a compressed window may integrate smoothly. Appetite aligns. Performance remains stable. Recovery unfolds predictably. The structure appears universally compatible. Yet this compatibility was contextual.

When workload increases without timing shift, the relationship changes. A promotion that extends cognitive load into evening hours, a training cycle that intensifies volume, or a new caregiving role that fragments sleep alters demand. If intake timing remains static, restoration must compete with expanded output. The margin that once absorbed fluctuation narrows. Performance may plateau quietly before baseline functioning changes.

Identical windows produce divergent outcomes because contexts diverge. One individual operates within moderate demand and ample sleep. Another navigates high stress density and reduced recovery opportunity. The feeding structure is identical; the energetic terrain is not.

Aging illustrates this terrain shift clearly. Recovery kinetics lengthen gradually. Sleep architecture evolves. The same timing pattern tolerated in earlier adulthood may compress margin later without visible intake change. Adaptive capacity changes over time. Structural integrity requires acknowledging that movement.

Demand timing matters alongside magnitude. High-output periods that align poorly with intake windows may compress restoration even when total demand is not extreme. When peak effort consistently precedes or follows prolonged fasting without adequate recovery opportunity, the system reallocates toward preservation rather than expansion. Ceiling narrows before baseline fails.

Proportional restoration dominance defines long-horizon stability. When restoration opportunity predominates relative to cumulative demand, the adaptive envelope expands or remains elastic. When mobilization consistently outweighs restoration—even subtly—compression unfolds gradually. The window itself is not causal; the proportion is.

Contextual integration looks different. When timing architecture acknowledges shifting demand—without ideological attachment to fixed boundaries—margin is preserved. Stability arises not from identical repetition but from relational coherence.

Flexibility signals structural intelligence because it reflects responsiveness to context. Rigid uniformity across changing terrain indicates detachment from proportion. Stability does not require uniformity; it requires alignment.

Tolerance is dynamic. What integrates during one life phase may compress during another. Workload, sleep, stress density, aging, and training cycles reshape the energetic landscape continuously. Fasting structure must therefore be interpreted as contextual architecture rather than fixed prescription.

Proportional alignment preserves ceiling by ensuring that intake timing and restoration opportunity remain commensurate with demand. Mismatch narrows ceiling first because the body prioritizes baseline survival over peak output. When alignment is maintained, variability tolerance remains broad. When alignment drifts, small perturbations produce disproportionate strain.

Stability is not achieved by enforcing identical windows regardless of environment. It is achieved by maintaining coherence between timing and evolving context. Early success does not guarantee permanent compatibility. Workload increases without timing adjustment alter proportion. Aging shifts recovery baseline. Life phases compress or expand margin.

Alignment is rarely dramatic. It is felt in the absence of friction. Sleep initiates without resistance. Hunger aligns predictably with intake windows. Peak output remains accessible without disproportionate effort. Minor schedule deviations do not destabilize mood or performance. These signals indicate proportion between intake timing and demand.

Misalignment appears first as subtle tension. Evening hunger intrudes into sleep onset. Morning performance requires more activation. High-output efforts feel accessible but less repeatable. Recovery extends slightly beyond expectation. None of these shifts indicate collapse. They indicate a narrowing envelope.

The body protects baseline survival before peak output. When proportion drifts, it trims capacity at the edges. Maximal effort declines before routine function fails. This trimming can be misinterpreted as lack of discipline or insufficient optimization. In reality, it reflects proportional reallocation.

Restoration dominance is the central stabilizer across contexts. When intake timing consistently allows recovery processes to bracket peak demand in a way that preserves sleep and stress modulation, adaptive capacity remains elastic. When mobilization repeatedly precedes restoration under compressed recovery windows, conservation becomes more likely.

Structural intelligence reflects responsiveness to terrain. It recognizes that identical architecture placed on evolving ground produces different load distributions. Structural identity, by contrast, attaches to form independent of function. Stability requires the former.

Ceiling preservation across time is the clearest indicator of alignment. When high-output capacity remains accessible despite contextual shifts, proportion is intact. When high output becomes progressively less repeatable under unchanged structure, terrain has moved.

Fasting stability is determined by proportional alignment between intake timing and evolving demand across contexts, not by adherence to a fixed window independent of environment.

Sex-Specific Adaptive Differences

Reproduction is not energetically neutral. It represents one of the most resource-intensive biological commitments an organism can undertake. The metabolic cost of gamete production, gestation, and potential lactation differs across sexes, and these differences shape how energy availability is interpreted.

Biological investment asymmetry begins at the level of reproductive strategy. Sperm production is continuous and relatively low in energetic cost compared with the cyclical preparation of an endometrium, ovulation, and the potential for gestation. Pregnancy requires sustained nutrient transfer, tissue expansion, and metabolic recalibration. Lactation extends this investment further. The energetic burden associated with reproduction is therefore not equivalent.

Because of this asymmetry, the reproductive axis functions as an environmental sensor. It interprets energy availability as a signal of whether expansion is proportionate to current conditions. When resources are abundant relative to demand, reproductive signaling remains robust. When availability narrows relative to workload or stress density, signaling may scale.

This scaling is proportional rather than pathological. The body prioritizes survival first and expansion second. Reproductive processes represent expansion. Under marginal availability, downscaling of reproductive signaling reflects conservation logic. It is not malfunction; it is adaptive prioritization.

Small deficits may register differently because thresholds differ. When the energetic cost of potential reproduction is high, signaling sensitivity increases. The body interprets subtle shifts in availability relative to demand as environmental information. This does not imply fragility. It reflects calibrated responsiveness to investment cost.

A subtle shift in menstrual cycle length under sustained marginal availability illustrates this proportional interpretation. An individual maintaining a compressed feeding window during a period of elevated workload may notice slight lengthening of cycle intervals over several months. Daily function remains intact. Performance appears stable. The shift represents environmental reading, not dysfunction. When restoration proportion increases, cycle length often normalizes gradually.

In contrast, stable adaptation under adequate proportion demonstrates robustness. An individual with balanced availability relative to demand may maintain consistent cycle patterns even with moderate fasting structure. The reproductive axis reads the environment as sufficient. Signaling remains coherent.

Male adaptive scaling often expresses differently. Because direct gestational investment is absent, the energetic threshold for reproductive downscaling may be higher. Testosterone levels may modulate under sustained marginal availability, yet small shifts may not produce immediate visible changes in reproductive capacity. The conservation logic still applies; its expression differs in magnitude and timing.

Energy signaling through the reproductive axis integrates multiple inputs: intake timing, total availability, stress load, sleep architecture, and workload. The axis does not respond to fasting alone but to the cumulative energetic landscape. Under proportionate alignment, signaling remains stable. Under sustained marginal conditions, scaling occurs.

This scaling may be subtle. Ovulatory timing may shift slightly. Basal temperature patterns may change modestly. These changes often precede overt performance compression. They reflect environmental assessment rather than structural collapse.

Reproductive signaling therefore serves as an environmental barometer. It interprets availability relative to demand and investment cost. Cost asymmetry between sexes shapes sensitivity thresholds, but the underlying logic is consistent: expansion proceeds when conditions support it.

Interpretation must remain contextual. A minor shift during intense workload and compressed recovery differs from an identical shift under stable conditions.

Reproductive permissiveness is not binary. It exists on a spectrum. The system does not switch abruptly from "on" to "off" in response to modest shifts in availability. Instead, amplitude adjusts. Signaling intensity can narrow before function disappears. Hormonal pulsatility may change subtly before overt cycle disruption appears. These gradations reflect continuous environmental interpretation rather than threshold collapse.

Energetic buffering capacity influences how long marginal availability can be tolerated without visible reproductive modulation. When gestational investment is possible, the organism maintains tighter surveillance over energy sufficiency. The cost of misjudgment is high. Entering a resource-intensive state under insufficient availability risks long-horizon instability. As a result, signaling often adjusts earlier in response to subtle shifts.

This earlier adjustment should not be interpreted as weakness. It represents anticipatory calibration. Systems with higher downstream cost of expansion often employ more sensitive upstream sensors. The logic mirrors other biological systems in which early detection preserves long-term stability.

Short-horizon tolerance can mask long-horizon scaling. An individual may maintain regular cycles during weeks of elevated demand and compressed intake. Over months, slight shifts accumulate. The modulation may remain minimal—slightly altered cycle length or reduced luteal phase duration—yet these shifts indicate cumulative interpretation rather than immediate crisis.

Stress load interacts strongly with this axis. Sleep disruption, psychological strain, and high workload amplify the environmental signal. Because reproductive permissiveness integrates the total energetic landscape rather than intake alone, fasting tolerance differs depending on cumulative load. Under stable sleep and moderate demand, compressed timing may integrate without modulation. Under stacked stress, identical structure may alter signaling thresholds.

Male reproductive signaling follows similar conservation logic but with different amplitude characteristics. Testosterone levels may adjust under prolonged marginal availability or high stress. However, because direct gestational investment does not occur, the urgency of scaling may differ. Modulation can still occur—libido shifts, subtle hormonal variation—but visible reproductive disruption may appear later relative to equivalent energetic strain.

Importantly, reproductive modulation often precedes overt performance compression. An individual may notice slight cycle irregularity before experiencing measurable strength plateau. This sequencing reflects prioritization hierarchy: expansion potential is assessed continuously and adjusted before baseline survival systems are compromised.

Energetic interpretation through the reproductive axis therefore functions as long-horizon risk management. It asks not whether the present moment is survivable, but whether sustained expansion is proportionate to environmental stability.

These differences in signaling thresholds do not imply categorical incompatibility with fasting. They illustrate that the same timing structure may produce distinct environmental readings depending on reproductive investment cost and cumulative load.

Energy availability is not measured consciously by the body; it is inferred through flux. The nervous system and endocrine network detect patterns of intake, expenditure, sleep, and stress across time. Pulsatile hormone signaling translates these patterns into modulation of metabolism, appetite, and reproductive readiness. Sensitivity to these signals varies, and the amplitude of response differs across individuals and, on average, between sexes.

Low energy availability is detected through multiple channels. Leptin reflects longer-horizon energy stores and recent intake. Thyroid hormones adjust metabolic rate relative to sustained availability. Cortisol and sympathetic tone signal stress density. These inputs converge, forming an integrated assessment of environmental sufficiency.

When availability narrows relative to demand, responses can manifest as appetite amplification, appetite suppression, metabolic rate modulation, or altered substrate use. The pattern is not uniform. It depends on context, body composition, and signaling thresholds.

In some individuals, compression of feeding windows under high workload produces noticeable appetite amplification. Hunger rises sharply near the end of the fasting interval. Evening intake becomes denser. The amplification reflects the body's attempt to restore proportion. In others, appetite may initially suppress under stress, only to rebound later when strain accumulates. These divergent responses illustrate variability in sensitivity.

On average, female physiology tends to exhibit earlier scaling under sustained marginal availability. Because reproductive investment carries higher energetic cost, environmental sufficiency thresholds may be interpreted with greater caution. Thyroid modulation may appear sooner relative to sustained proportion shifts. Leptin signaling may exert stronger influence on reproductive axis calibration. These differences represent amplitude variation rather than categorical distinction.

Male physiology may tolerate marginal availability longer before visible reproductive modulation occurs. Appetite patterns may shift differently. Testosterone may scale gradually without overt reproductive disruption. However, under sufficient stress stacking and prolonged marginal intake, scaling still occurs. The amplitude and timing differ, not the underlying logic.

Fat oxidation patterns also differ on average. Females often demonstrate greater reliance on lipid substrates at comparable activity intensities. This buffering capacity may support endurance under certain conditions but does not eliminate sensitivity to sustained low availability.

Body composition interacts with these dynamics. Higher fat mass can provide short-term energetic buffering, moderating leptin decline and metabolic scaling. Lower fat mass narrows that buffer, increasing sensitivity to compression.

An individual with moderate body fat and proportionate intake may maintain stable adaptation under a compressed window during moderate workload. Appetite remains predictable. Sleep is intact. Performance holds steady. The same structure applied to an individual with lower body fat under high training load may produce earlier appetite volatility and thyroid modulation. Context and composition alter amplitude.

Sleep interaction further shapes sensitivity. Sleep loss amplifies stress signaling and reduces leptin responsiveness. Under identical feeding windows, an individual sleeping seven to eight hours may maintain stable signaling, while one sleeping five to six hours experiences amplified hunger and mood variability. Sensitivity layers across systems.

Stress stacking magnifies amplitude. Occupational strain, emotional demand, and training volume collectively increase signal intensity. Under stacked stress, pulsatile hormone signaling may become more volatile. Appetite cues intensify or become erratic. Scaling may occur earlier than predicted by intake alone.

Short-horizon adaptation can mask long-horizon scaling. In the first weeks of compression, catecholamine elevation may enhance alertness. Fat oxidation may increase transiently. Appetite may feel controlled. Over months, however, if availability remains marginal relative to demand, thyroid modulation and reproductive scaling may become evident. The early phase reflects acute adjustment; the later phase reflects cumulative interpretation.

Individual variability within sexes is substantial. Genetic differences, prior dieting history, sleep patterns, body composition, and psychological stress all influence sensitivity. Some women maintain stable signaling under substantial workload and compressed feeding. Some men exhibit early scaling under moderate marginal availability. Average trends do not determine individual response.

An example clarifies amplitude differences. Two individuals adopt identical six-hour feeding windows under similar workloads. One, a female with lower body fat and high training volume, experiences earlier appetite amplification and subtle cycle variability after several months. The other, a male with moderate body fat and moderate training, maintains stable appetite and performance longer before noticing scaling. The difference reflects amplitude and threshold, not categorical suitability.

Differential sensitivity also explains why identical fasting windows feel subjectively different. One individual reports calm focus and stable hunger. Another reports heightened irritability and evening appetite spikes. The structure is identical; signal interpretation differs.

Energy buffering through body composition modifies detection thresholds. Greater stored energy can delay leptin decline under compression, smoothing early adaptation. Lower stores narrow margin, increasing responsiveness. This does not imply superiority of one state; it illustrates proportional detection logic.

Differential energy sensitivity therefore represents variation in how adaptive scaling is expressed. The amplitude and timing of response differ according to reproductive investment cost, body composition, stress density, and sleep integrity. The underlying mechanism remains consistent: environmental interpretation through integrated signaling.

Differential sensitivity to fasting reflects amplitude variation in adaptive scaling rather than categorical suitability or unsuitability for timing-based feeding structures.

Hormonal systems rarely change in straight lines. They scale gradually across a range and then, at certain points, appear to shift more abruptly. This pattern reflects threshold behavior. Beneath visible inflection lies cumulative proportional strain that has crossed a detection boundary.

Adaptation often unfolds quietly at first. Under modest compression of availability relative to demand, pulsatile rhythms remain intact. Hormone pulses continue at predictable intervals, even if amplitude narrows slightly. Thyroid output may taper modestly. Reproductive signaling may soften without overt disruption. The organism remains functionally stable.

Gradual scaling can persist for months without obvious markers. An individual training regularly while maintaining compressed intake may experience slightly longer recovery times yet maintain performance. Sleep feels somewhat lighter. Appetite fluctuates modestly. These changes distribute across domains and do not immediately converge into a visible event.

Threshold behavior emerges when cumulative load—availability compression, stress density, sleep reduction—crosses an internal detection point. At that point, signaling patterns can shift more visibly. What seemed stable may alter within a short interval, not because the system failed suddenly, but because the cumulative burden reached an inflection.

Cortisol and thyroid signaling illustrate this interplay. Under sustained stress and marginal availability, cortisol may remain modestly elevated for longer portions of the day. Thyroid signaling may downscale gradually to conserve energy. When sleep compression persists alongside high workload, the interaction between these signals can reach a threshold where metabolic scaling becomes more apparent. The shift may feel abrupt, but the groundwork was incremental.

In women, reproductive axis inflection often provides a visible marker of threshold crossing. A cycle that had lengthened slightly over several months may suddenly skip or delay more noticeably. The change appears sudden. Yet prior months likely included subtle amplitude narrowing in pulsatile gonadotropin signaling. The threshold was crossed when cumulative load exceeded proportional tolerance.

In men, testosterone modulation may follow a similar nonlinear pattern. Under prolonged marginal availability and high stress, testosterone levels may decline gradually. Performance plateau may precede noticeable change in libido or mood. When cumulative strain persists, the decline may become more pronounced within a short interval. Again, the apparent abruptness masks extended scaling.

Loss of amplitude differs from loss of rhythm. In early scaling, pulses remain rhythmic but smaller. After threshold crossing, rhythm itself may become irregular. Sleep disruption accelerates this shift because nightly consolidation supports pulse coherence. Without adequate sleep, pulsatile patterns destabilize more readily.

Stress stacking amplifies threshold dynamics. Moderate availability compression alone may not trigger inflection. Combined with high training load, emotional strain, and sleep loss, the cumulative burden crosses detection thresholds more quickly. The endocrine system interprets the environment as less supportive of expansion and scales accordingly.

Early signals are often missed because they distribute across systems. Slight appetite volatility, marginal mood shifts, subtle recovery delay—each seems trivial in isolation. Only when multiple small shifts converge does the inflection become visible. The plateau that preceded visible endocrine change often represents early scaling that had not yet crossed threshold.

One example of gradual scaling involves a female endurance athlete maintaining compressed intake during moderate training. Over months, cycles lengthen by a few days. Performance remains steady. After adding higher-intensity sessions and travel stress, a cycle is delayed more substantially. The delay feels abrupt, yet the earlier lengthening signaled cumulative narrowing.

A male example might involve prolonged heavy training under compressed feeding. Strength gains plateau subtly. Sleep becomes lighter. Testosterone modulation may remain modest until additional workload or stress crosses threshold, after which fatigue deepens and mood shifts more noticeably. The apparent abruptness reflects accumulated proportional strain.

Thresholds vary individually. Genetic predisposition, body composition, sleep resilience, and stress buffering capacity shape detection points. Two individuals under identical intake and workload may exhibit different inflection timing. Sensitivity is not uniform.

The nonlinear nature of hormonal thresholds underscores that adaptation is rarely binary. Stability can mask gradual scaling until cumulative factors converge. When visible shifts occur, they represent expression of prior integration rather than isolated events.

Hormonal thresholds therefore function as nonlinear expressions of cumulative proportional strain, revealing inflection points that arise from sustained context rather than abrupt dysfunction.

When two individuals adopt the same fasting window, the visible structure is identical. The internal response rarely is. Appetite, mood stability, performance trajectory, and recovery patterns diverge not because one structure is correct and the other flawed, but because adaptive responses cluster differently across biological and contextual variables.

Appetite provides one of the clearest examples. Under compressed feeding, some individuals experience rapid appetite stabilization. Hunger concentrates predictably within the window and remains muted outside it. Others encounter increasing volatility: sharp late-day hunger spikes, alternating suppression and amplification, or subtle shifts in satiety recognition. These patterns reflect differences in signal prioritization, not discipline.

Mood and stress resilience often diverge as well. Under identical compression, one person may report heightened clarity and emotional steadiness for weeks. Another may experience increasing irritability as workload accumulates. Both remain adherent. The divergence lies in how stress signaling integrates with energy availability and sleep architecture.

Performance ceilings also behave differently. In some men, early adaptation to fasting under moderate training appears robust. Fat oxidation increases, perceived endurance improves, and training feels efficient. Weeks later, under intensified workload, the shift can become more pronounced—strength plateau, recovery lag, and mood compression appearing with larger amplitude once scaling begins.

In contrast, many women display earlier but more protective scaling under similar conditions. Appetite may become more noticeable sooner. Subtle recovery adjustments appear earlier. Rather than experiencing large later shifts, adaptation moderates earlier. The earlier signal can function as protective recalibration that preserves long-horizon stability.

These are probabilistic tendencies rather than rules. Variability within sexes exceeds average differences between them. Individual body composition, sleep quality, psychological stress, and prior metabolic history shape response clusters more strongly than sex alone.

Consider two endurance athletes—one male, one female—adopting identical six-hour feeding windows during moderate training. Initially, the male athlete reports strong training output and stable mood. The female athlete notices slightly increased hunger and minor recovery shifts within the first months. As training volume increases, the male athlete experiences a more abrupt performance plateau and pronounced fatigue. The female athlete, having scaled earlier, maintains steadier performance.

The divergence reflects timing and amplitude differences in adaptive scaling.

A reverse pattern also occurs. A female strength athlete with moderate body fat and consistent sleep may integrate compressed feeding with minimal volatility. A male counterpart under high stress and lower body fat may experience early appetite instability and plateau. The expected pattern reverses because context overrides averages.

Fat oxidation differences contribute to these divergent patterns. On average, women rely more heavily on lipid substrates at comparable intensities. This endurance bias may support steady-state performance under moderate compression. However, glycogen recovery dynamics differ as well. In high-intensity or power-oriented contexts, restoration timing may influence adaptation differently across individuals.

Energy buffering via body composition modifies these effects. Higher fat mass can buffer short-horizon compression, smoothing appetite and thyroid signaling shifts. Lower reserves narrow margin, increasing sensitivity regardless of sex. Sleep sensitivity compounds variability. Individuals whose sleep degrades quickly under stress may exhibit earlier scaling independent of reproductive investment patterns.

Anecdotal comparisons can mislead because they isolate visible structure while ignoring pattern clusters. Two people following identical timing may attribute differences to willpower or inherent suitability. In reality, signal prioritization, buffering capacity, stress density, and sleep architecture interact to produce divergent outcomes.

Men often display later but more pronounced scaling when cumulative load exceeds threshold, reflecting larger amplitude once protective mechanisms engage. Women often exhibit earlier modulation that tempers strain before larger shifts occur. Yet these are tendencies, not absolutes. Individual context frequently overrides sex-based averages.

Divergent adaptive response patterns under identical fasting structures arise from clustered biological and contextual variables rather than categorical suitability, reflecting probabilistic sex-specific scaling tendencies within broader individual variability.

Sex-based differences in fasting response are often discussed as categorical rules. One sex is said to tolerate compression better; the other is described as more vulnerable. These summaries oversimplify what is, in practice, a question of amplitude, timing, and context.

Adaptive responses unfold along gradients. On average, some individuals may exhibit earlier modulation in reproductive or thyroid signaling. Others may demonstrate later but larger shifts once cumulative load exceeds threshold. These patterns reflect differences in scaling dynamics rather than differences in suitability.

Categorical rules fail because they ignore context. Sleep architecture, stress density, workload, body composition, and life phase frequently override average tendencies. A woman with stable sleep, moderate workload, and proportionate intake may integrate compressed feeding for years without instability. A man with high stress, fragmented sleep, and marginal availability may destabilize under the same structure. The window does not determine the outcome; the environment does.

Probabilistic trends describe populations, not individuals. They cannot prescribe or prohibit fasting for a specific person. Individual threshold variability remains wide. Two people of the same sex, similar age, and similar body composition may diverge dramatically in tolerance under identical timing structures because stress integration, sleep resilience, and prior metabolic history differ.

A categorical recommendation that "women should avoid fasting" or "men handle fasting better" collapses this complexity into slogan. Consider a female endurance athlete in a stable training block with consistent sleep and balanced availability. Compressed feeding integrates without volatility. Now consider a male professional under chronic stress and poor sleep adopting the same window. Mood variability and recovery compression appear within months. The categorical rule misleads both.

Internal signal stability offers more informative guidance than external structure. When sleep remains coherent, appetite predictable, mood stable, and performance ceiling intact, adaptation is likely proportionate. When volatility increases—sleep drift, erratic hunger, plateau with rising effort—the mismatch lies not in sex category but in contextual alignment.

Anecdotal success stories often distort interpretation. An individual may report dramatic early benefit under fasting, attributing improvement to inherent compatibility. Over time, life phase shifts—training escalation, aging recovery changes, increased stress—alter integration. Early success does not guarantee long-horizon stability. Conversely, someone who struggles initially may stabilize as workload moderates or sleep improves.

Social comparison compounds distortion. Observing another person thrive under identical timing invites assumptions of universal applicability. Yet unseen variables—body composition buffering, sleep consistency, stress load—shape response amplitude. Comparing structures without comparing contexts leads to inaccurate conclusions.

Adaptive range matters more than protocol. A wide adaptive range permits fluctuation without volatility. A narrow range magnifies small mismatches. Sex-based averages may influence scaling amplitude, but adaptive range is constructed through integrated proportion across cycles.

Life phase transitions further illustrate non-binary adaptation. A woman may integrate fasting comfortably in one decade and experience earlier scaling in another as recovery kinetics change. A man may tolerate compression during sedentary years and encounter instability when training volume intensifies. Context evolves continuously.

Energy buffering differences influence perception. Individuals with greater stored energy may display smoother early adaptation. Those with lower reserves may register marginal availability sooner. These differences cross sex lines and complicate categorical narratives.

An example of categorical advice failing can be seen in a male athlete encouraged to fast because "men respond well." Under heavy training and poor sleep, he experiences early plateau and mood compression. Meanwhile, a female colleague integrates the same window during a moderate training phase without issue. The rule predicted the opposite.

Internal signal tracking reveals mismatch more reliably than external comparison. An individual noticing gradual sleep drift and increased appetite volatility despite strict adherence is not observing failure of discipline but evidence of contextual misalignment.

Both sexes can integrate fasting well when proportion aligns with demand and recovery. Both sexes can destabilize under sustained mismatch. The difference lies in scaling dynamics and context, not categorical compatibility.

Sex-specific adaptive differences therefore represent contextual scaling phenomena within broader human metabolic architecture, expressing amplitude and timing variation rather than fixed rules about fasting suitability.

Aging and Narrowing Recovery Margins

Muscle tissue is in constant turnover. Protein synthesis and protein breakdown occur simultaneously, adjusting to mechanical demand, hormonal signaling, sleep quality, and energy availability. Across decades of life, this turnover remains active, but the amplitude and speed of certain processes shift gradually.

In early adulthood, anabolic signaling in response to training is typically robust. Mechanical tension triggers satellite cell activation and coordinated protein synthesis. The amplitude of synthesis following a stimulus is relatively high, and recovery kinetics are comparatively rapid. Sleep architecture supports this cycle through nocturnal repair processes, and the hormonal environment generally amplifies adaptive response.

By midlife and beyond, the fundamental machinery remains intact, yet certain parameters change. Satellite cell responsiveness may decline modestly. The amplitude of protein synthesis following a given stimulus may be slightly lower. Recovery kinetics—how quickly muscle returns to baseline readiness after stress—often lengthen. These shifts are gradual rather than abrupt.

The slowing of recovery kinetics does not imply loss of adaptability. It reflects recalibration of bandwidth. When recovery takes longer, the margin between stimulus and restoration narrows under identical structural demands. A training stimulus tolerated easily at 25 may require slightly more proportional restoration at 55 to produce the same adaptation.

Energy availability interacts with this dynamic. In younger decades, modest compression of intake timing may integrate without obvious strain, particularly if sleep is stable and stress load moderate. In later decades, the same compression layered onto identical training intensity may subtly reduce recovery margin. Muscle soreness may persist longer. Performance peaks may require more deliberate restoration to reappear.

Consider a 25-year-old and a 55-year-old following identical fasting windows while performing comparable resistance training routines. Initially, both may progress. The younger individual experiences rapid recovery between sessions. Protein synthesis amplitude peaks and resolves efficiently. The older individual also adapts, but recovery lag is slightly longer. If intake timing compresses the restoration window, cumulative strain may appear earlier in the older athlete—not because training is inappropriate, but because bandwidth is narrower.

Hormonal environment shifts across decades contribute to this pattern. Testosterone levels in men and estrogen levels in women change gradually with age, altering the anabolic milieu. Growth hormone secretion patterns evolve. These changes influence the amplitude of repair signaling without eliminating it.

Sleep plays a central role in this interaction. Deep sleep phases support tissue repair and anabolic signaling. With age, sleep may become lighter or more fragmented. When fasting compresses intake and overlaps with stress or late-night workload, sleep quality may degrade slightly. In younger decades this may be absorbed without visible impact. In later decades the same disruption may slow recovery enough to narrow margin.

Stress tolerance also shifts. The cumulative stress density that could once be absorbed without performance drift may now require proportionate restoration to maintain output. Recovery buffer—the surplus capacity that allows adaptation beyond baseline—reduces gradually.

Plateau appears differently at 25 versus 55. In early adulthood, plateau often reflects the need for increased stimulus or strategic variation. In later decades, plateau may reflect interaction between stimulus, recovery, and availability. Escalation of stimulus without proportional restoration may compress capacity rather than expand it.

An example illustrates recovery lag accumulation. A 55-year-old lifter maintains a six-hour feeding window and trains intensely four times per week. For several months, progress continues. Gradually, soreness persists longer between sessions. Strength increases slow. Sleep becomes slightly lighter. The structure remains identical to earlier years, yet recovery buffer has narrowed. Minor adjustments in proportional restoration—without abandoning training or fasting—can preserve output and reduce lag.

Moderate alignment changes can maintain stability without dramatic restructuring. Slight widening of the recovery window around high-demand sessions, improved sleep consistency, or moderated training density may preserve anabolic signaling amplitude sufficiently to sustain adaptation. These adjustments represent alignment rather than retreat.

Variability remains wide. Some individuals in their fifties and sixties demonstrate remarkable recovery capacity, particularly when sleep, stress, and availability align proportionately. Others experience earlier narrowing. Aging does not eliminate adaptability; it recalibrates the conditions under which adaptability expresses.

Preservation becomes the primary adaptation in later decades. Rather than pursuing maximal expansion, architecture often shifts toward maintaining ceiling and protecting margin. This preservation is not resignation. It reflects intelligent allocation of recovery resources relative to demand.

Identical fasting windows that felt neutral in early adulthood may compress margin later because recovery kinetics have slowed and hormonal amplitude has shifted. The solution is not abandonment of structure but recognition of evolving context.

Aging therefore represents gradual narrowing of recovery bandwidth that requires proportional alignment between stimulus, intake timing, and restoration rather than withdrawal from fasting or training altogether.

Across decades, insulin signaling does not disappear; it redistributes. Sensitivity shifts among tissues, storage capacity changes subtly, and the timing of glucose handling becomes more context-dependent. These alterations are not failures of regulation but recalibrations within a changing physiological landscape.

Skeletal muscle functions as a primary glucose sink. In early adulthood, relatively high muscle mass and strong contractile responsiveness allow efficient peripheral uptake following meals. Glycogen storage amplitude—the total capacity to store carbohydrate within muscle—tends to be robust. Postprandial excursions are often modest because disposal capacity is high.

With aging, gradual changes in body composition influence this dynamic. Muscle mass may decline modestly across decades, particularly if training stimulus and recovery proportion are not aligned. Concurrently, fat mass may redistribute, with greater tendency toward central or visceral accumulation in some individuals. This redistribution alters relative tissue sensitivity patterns. Hepatic insulin responsiveness may remain intact or even increase, while peripheral muscle sensitivity may decrease slightly if muscle mass declines.

The result is not categorical dysfunction but altered partitioning. A given meal may produce a slightly higher or more prolonged glucose excursion at 65 than at 30, even when total intake is identical. Reduced glycogen capacity in muscle narrows the amplitude of storage, particularly when recovery between high-output days is compressed. Muscle still responds, but its buffering capacity is smaller.

Hepatic glucose regulation becomes more prominent in this context. The liver balances endogenous production and storage. Sleep quality, stress density, and circadian rhythm strongly influence this process.

With lighter or fragmented sleep—a pattern more common in later decades—overnight glucose regulation may shift subtly, increasing fasting glucose variability without indicating structural pathology.

Consider a 30-year-old and a 65-year-old following identical eight-hour feeding windows with similar activity levels. Both may feel stable during fasting hours. Catecholamine support maintains alertness, and lipolysis proceeds effectively. However, when the feeding window opens, the younger individual may replenish muscle glycogen more rapidly and return to baseline sooner. The older individual may experience slightly longer postprandial elevation and slower glycogen restoration, particularly if muscle mass is reduced. The difference is quantitative rather than categorical.

These shifts influence fasting tolerance indirectly. Many older adults report feeling metabolically steady during fasting intervals—sometimes even more comfortable than in youth. Lipid oxidation capacity often remains strong. However, recovery from intense training or high cognitive demand may lag when intake is compressed. The fasting interval itself may feel neutral, yet restoration within the feeding window may not fully replenish prior demand, especially if glycogen capacity is smaller.

Energy partitioning patterns also evolve. A slightly higher proportion of incoming energy may be directed toward hepatic storage or adipose tissue if muscle disposal capacity is reduced. This does not imply inevitability of fat gain; rather, it reflects altered distribution. Resistance training and preserved muscle mass can maintain peripheral disposal capacity well into later decades, illustrating the wide variability across individuals.

Circadian influences become increasingly relevant. Glucose tolerance often varies more distinctly by time of day in older adults. Late feeding may produce more pronounced excursions than earlier intake under identical conditions. Sleep disruption interacts with this pattern, amplifying variability. Stress hormones—particularly when elevated chronically—can increase hepatic glucose output, subtly shifting postprandial dynamics.

Recovery lag under compressed intake illustrates how redistribution affects experience. A 65-year-old engaging in resistance training within a narrow feeding window may initially progress. Over time, performance peaks flatten slightly. Glycogen replenishment lags behind stimulus. The window remains unchanged, but adaptive range narrows. Widening recovery proportion—even modestly—often restores smoother oscillation without abandoning structure.

Stable metabolic flexibility in later decades is common when muscle mass is preserved, sleep coherent, and workload proportionate. Many individuals in their sixties demonstrate effective substrate switching, smooth fasting tolerance, and stable postprandial handling. Adaptive range narrows relative to earlier decades but does not vanish.

Variability remains broad. Genetics, lifelong training history, body composition, and stress integration shape redistribution patterns. Some individuals maintain peripheral sensitivity well into older age. Others experience earlier shifts. Age modifies probability, not destiny.

Identical fasting windows therefore behave differently at 30 and 65 because tissue capacity, storage amplitude, circadian regulation, and recovery kinetics have shifted. Timing structure remains neutral. Its integration depends on the evolving distribution of metabolic flexibility across tissues.

This narrowing can produce an interesting contrast in subjective experience. Many older adults report feeling metabolically steady during fasting intervals. Lipid oxidation remains effective, appetite may be calm, and cognitive clarity stable. Yet restoration after high demand may lag quietly. The fasting state itself does not feel destabilizing, but cumulative restoration within the feeding window may not fully match prior expenditure when storage amplitude is reduced. The result is gradual flattening rather than abrupt disruption.

Sleep quality interacts with this redistribution. Lighter or more fragmented sleep can increase hepatic glucose output modestly and reduce peripheral insulin sensitivity transiently. In a system with narrower glycogen bandwidth, this adds incremental strain. None of these shifts indicate inevitable decline. They illustrate how adaptive range narrows gradually, requiring proportional alignment between intake timing, workload, and recovery opportunity to maintain stability.

Adaptive flexibility persists across decades, but its oscillation bandwidth contracts. The same fasting structure that once allowed wide metabolic swings may now require slightly greater restoration density to preserve ceiling. The governing principle remains proportion rather than abandonment.

Aging-related insulin shifts therefore represent redistribution of metabolic flexibility and disposal capacity across organs and contexts, requiring proportional alignment with muscle mass, sleep integrity, and workload rather than signaling inevitable dysfunction.

Sleep is not a passive state. It is a coordinated anabolic interval during which neural repair, glycogen restoration, immune modulation, and hormone pulse consolidation occur in synchronized sequence. Across decades, the architecture of this interval shifts gradually. These shifts do not eliminate restorative capacity, but they alter the density and timing of repair.

Slow-wave sleep—the deepest stage associated with physical restoration—tends to decrease modestly with age. REM distribution may shift, and sleep fragmentation becomes more common. Many adults notice earlier chronotype drift, with natural sleep onset and waking occurring earlier than in younger years. These changes unfold incrementally rather than abruptly.

Slow-wave sleep acts as an amplifier of recovery. Growth hormone pulses cluster during deeper stages, supporting tissue repair and metabolic recalibration. Glycogen restoration in muscle and liver is partly sleep-dependent, as nocturnal parasympathetic dominance facilitates storage and cellular repair. When slow-wave duration shortens, the window for concentrated repair compresses. Recovery remains possible, but consolidation becomes more sensitive to disruption.

REM sleep contributes to neural integration and emotional regulation. Changes in REM distribution can subtly influence cognitive resilience and stress processing. Fragmentation—brief awakenings or lighter transitions between stages—reduces continuity of recovery. The body still cycles through stages, yet the efficiency of consolidation may decrease.

Interaction with cortisol rhythm becomes more apparent under these conditions. In younger adults, robust sleep architecture buffers modest fluctuations in stress load. Cortisol peaks and troughs maintain predictable amplitude. In later decades, lighter sleep can allow greater nocturnal cortisol variability. This does not indicate dysfunction, but it can alter morning energy perception and glucose regulation patterns.

Fasting timing intersects with this architecture. A feeding window that extends later into the evening may feel neutral at 30, when slow-wave density remains high and fragmentation minimal. At 65, the same timing may overlap more closely with the body's earlier chronotype and lighter sleep pattern. Postprandial metabolic activity near bedtime can subtly delay sleep onset or increase fragmentation, reducing consolidation of repair. The difference lies not in morality of timing but in evolving sleep physiology.

Consider a 35-year-old and a 65-year-old following an identical feeding schedule that ends at 9:00 p.m. Both maintain consistent training routines. The younger adult falls asleep quickly and enters slow-wave sleep with minimal interruption. The older adult, whose natural chronotype now favors earlier sleep onset, experiences delayed sleep initiation and lighter first-cycle sleep. Recovery kinetics the following day diverge slightly. The feeding structure is unchanged; the architecture of sleep is not.

Sleep fragmentation can compound recovery lag. A 60-year-old engaging in resistance training while maintaining a compressed feeding window may initially progress. Over months, brief nocturnal awakenings increase. Muscle soreness persists longer, and training output plateaus subtly. The cumulative effect of lighter sleep narrows the margin available for adaptation, even though daily energy intake remains stable.

Chronotype drift can also create alignment opportunities. An individual in later decades who naturally feels alert earlier in the day may find that earlier feeding aligns more comfortably with endogenous rhythm. This alignment reduces nocturnal metabolic activity and supports consolidated sleep. The interaction demonstrates that timing integration is relational rather than fixed.

Fasting itself may feel metabolically neutral. Lipid oxidation remains intact, and subjective clarity may persist. Yet lighter sleep can compound strain when high training volume or cognitive load coexist with compressed intake. The fasting interval is not inherently destabilizing; rather, reduced recovery consolidation amplifies any mismatch between demand and restoration.

Stress tolerance often narrows subtly with lighter sleep. Emotional perturbations or workload spikes that were once absorbed without noticeable lag may now extend into subsequent days. Recovery from intense training sessions may require slightly more time. These shifts represent recalibration of adaptive range, not elimination of capacity.

Variability remains wide. Some individuals maintain deep, consolidated sleep into later decades and demonstrate strong recovery under diverse timing structures. Others experience earlier fragmentation and require closer alignment between feeding window and chronotype to preserve margin. Genetic predisposition, lifelong sleep patterns, and stress exposure all influence trajectory.

Adaptability persists throughout the lifespan. Sleep architecture shifts gradually, but repair mechanisms remain active. Muscle and neural tissue continue to respond to stimulus. The key difference lies in the density of recovery opportunity within a given night. When slow-wave and REM consolidation narrow, proportional alignment between demand, intake timing, and sleep rhythm becomes more influential.

Identical feeding windows therefore interact differently with sleep at 30 and 65 because recovery consolidation windows have shifted. The structure itself remains neutral. Its impact depends on the evolving architecture of sleep and stress integration.

This narrowing of consolidation bandwidth interacts with the redistribution of metabolic flexibility described earlier. If muscle glycogen amplitude is modestly reduced and nocturnal restoration slightly less dense, the system has fewer opportunities to replenish fully between high-demand days. Oscillation between depletion and repletion becomes tighter. In younger decades, wide slow-wave windows and higher glycogen capacity allow greater fluctuation without visible strain. In later decades, identical oscillations approach the edge of available bandwidth more quickly.

An important nuance emerges here. Many older adults report that fasting itself feels easier than in youth. Appetite may be calmer. Energy may feel stable. Lipid oxidation remains effective. Yet adaptation to high-intensity training or cumulative stress may slow. The subjective stability of the fasting interval does not necessarily reflect the density of nocturnal repair. Strain accumulates quietly at the level of recovery consolidation rather than during fasting hours themselves.

Sleep fragmentation also alters stress integration. Brief awakenings increase sympathetic activation even if total sleep duration remains similar. When this pattern repeats across weeks, cortisol rhythm may flatten slightly overnight. The following day begins with slightly reduced recovery reserve. Under compressed feeding, the system must mobilize and restore within tighter margins. No single day signals collapse, but the aggregate narrows adaptive elasticity.

None of these shifts eliminate adaptability. They reduce the amplitude of recovery oscillation available per cycle. When workload, feeding timing, and sleep architecture align proportionately, stability persists. When misalignment persists across cycles, compression becomes visible first in ceiling reduction rather than baseline failure.

Aging-related sleep shifts therefore represent gradual narrowing of recovery consolidation windows, requiring proportional alignment with feeding timing and workload rather than abandonment of fasting as a structural tool.

Timing architecture does not exist in isolation. It rests within a broader adaptive bandwidth that evolves gradually across decades. As recovery kinetics shift, sleep consolidates differently, and energy partitioning recalibrates, identical fasting structures interact with a changing internal landscape. What once felt expansive may later feel compressive—not because the structure has changed, but because the margin around it has narrowed.

In early adulthood, adaptive bandwidth is typically wide. Oscillation amplitude between fed and fasted states is strong, recovery consolidation is dense, and stress buffering capacity is comparatively high. Misalignment between demand and intake timing can persist for extended periods before visible compression appears. Plateau, when it occurs, often reflects stimulus saturation or behavioral drift rather than recovery limitation.

As decades progress, adaptive bandwidth narrows gradually. Oscillation remains present, but amplitude may be slightly reduced. Recovery windows become more sensitive to disruption. Stress density accumulates through career progression, caregiving responsibilities, and environmental load. The architecture of preservation begins to outweigh the architecture of expansion.

Identical fasting timing that once supported expansion may later compress margin under the same workload. Consider a 30-year-old and a 60-year-old following the same compressed feeding window while engaging in regular resistance training. The younger adult tolerates occasional late nights, variable stress, and high training intensity with little performance drift. The older adult initially adapts similarly, but subtle recovery lag accumulates. Strength gains plateau sooner. Sleep fragmentation compounds strain. The window remains unchanged; adaptive bandwidth has shifted.

Preservation becomes the primary adaptation—not as concession, but as intelligent recalibration. Ceiling retention requires proportional alignment between demand and restoration. Where expansion once required little adjustment, maintaining ceiling now depends on context integration.

Training cycles interact differently with timing across decades. In younger adults, peak training phases layered onto compressed feeding may produce robust adaptation. In later decades, peak demand without proportional recovery may narrow oscillation amplitude and reduce ceiling. Timing structure is not inherently incompatible with intensity; rather, its integration must reflect the evolving relationship between stimulus and restoration.

Plateau interpretation changes accordingly. At 30, plateau often signals need for novel stimulus or increased load. At 60, plateau may signal recovery bandwidth saturation rather than insufficient effort. Escalation strategies—further compression of the feeding window or intensification of training—may behave differently under narrowed bandwidth. What once expanded capacity may now compress it.

Structural inertia can produce mismatch. An individual who successfully maintained a particular fasting architecture for decades may attach identity to that structure even as context shifts. Career promotion increases stress density. Caregiving responsibilities fragment sleep. Training intensity remains unchanged. The structure that once aligned smoothly now subtly narrows margin. Plateau appears, yet interpretation defaults to "not enough intensity" rather than contextual recalibration.

A modest alignment shift can preserve output without dismantling architecture. Slight redistribution of demand relative to recovery, earlier alignment with chronotype drift, or moderated peak intensity during high-stress phases can restore oscillation amplitude sufficiently to maintain ceiling. The structure persists; its integration adapts.

Younger adults often tolerate misalignment longer because surplus bandwidth buffers volatility. Recovery lag remains minimal, and oscillation amplitude compensates for timing compression. Older adults require tighter proportional alignment because recovery margin is smaller and stress accumulation interacts more readily with feeding structure. This does not imply fragility. It reflects evolved efficiency and recalibrated resource allocation.

Energy buffering shifts across decades as body composition and metabolic partitioning evolve. Smaller glycogen capacity, altered muscle mass, and redistributed adipose tissue influence how feeding timing interacts with demand. Oscillation remains, but its amplitude becomes more context-sensitive. Escalation strategies that once felt adaptive may now reduce flexibility if recovery is not proportionately restored.

Identity attachment to structure can obscure this shift. A long-held fasting pattern becomes equated with discipline or stability. When plateau or subtle compression appears, the impulse may be to intensify adherence rather than examine contextual bandwidth. Structural inertia preserves familiarity but may conflict with evolving physiology.

Adaptability persists throughout life. Oscillation does not disappear. Muscle continues to respond to stimulus. Metabolic flexibility remains accessible. The difference lies in margin and amplitude. Younger decades allow greater deviation before compression appears. Later decades reward proportional alignment more immediately.

Variability across individuals remains substantial. Some sixty-year-olds maintain recovery bandwidth comparable to younger adults due to preserved muscle mass, coherent sleep, and moderate stress density. Some thirty-year-olds exhibit early compression under high stress and misaligned timing. Age modifies probability and sensitivity, not capacity itself.

Timing architecture across decades therefore becomes less about expansion and more about preserving ceiling within narrowing adaptive bandwidth. The window itself remains neutral. Its impact depends on how well it integrates with evolving recovery capacity, stress density, and life-phase demands.

Intermittent Fasting as a Contextual Tool

Intermittent fasting is a structure. It is a way of organizing time. It arranges feeding and fasting intervals into a recognizable pattern. Beyond that, it carries no inherent moral weight, no guaranteed outcome, and no automatic direction. Structure is not result. It is architecture within which results may—or may not—emerge.

Confusion begins when structure is mistaken for outcome. Compression of eating opportunity can feel productive. Tolerated hunger can feel like forward movement. Visible restraint carries psychological weight. Yet metabolic systems respond not to effort or identity, but to proportion, recovery, and cumulative alignment. A feeding window does not override physiology; it interacts with it.

Escalation often masquerades as progress. A plateau appears. The window tightens. The interval extends. The logic seems straightforward: more compression should amplify the effect. Yet escalation narrows adaptive bandwidth when recovery margin is already limited. What once felt expansive can become compressive through intensity alone.

Escalation drift illustrates this subtle shift. An individual begins with a moderate feeding structure and experiences smooth integration—stable energy, coherent sleep, preserved performance. Over time, progress slows. The interpretation defaults to insufficiency. The window compresses incrementally. Recovery narrows. Sleep fragments slightly. Performance plateaus further. The architecture remains intact, but oscillation amplitude contracts. Escalation does not produce expansion; it produces compression.

Neutrality protects adaptability because it permits recalibration without ideological resistance. When fasting is held as a tool rather than an identity, adjustments become architectural rather than emotional. Structure can widen or narrow according to context without threatening self-concept. Adaptive bandwidth is preserved because rigidity does not amplify stress.

Stable integration looks different. A person adopts a feeding pattern that aligns with workload and recovery capacity. Sleep remains coherent. Training oscillates without ceiling loss. Stress fluctuations are absorbed without volatility. The window persists not because it is defended, but because it fits. When life phase shifts—career demand increases, caregiving alters sleep, training intensity rises—the structure adjusts proportionally. Oscillation remains recoverable.

Plateau is frequently misread. It can signal completion of adaptation rather than insufficiency. In a neutral framework, plateau invites assessment of proportional alignment rather than automatic intensification. Sometimes stability is the correct outcome. Expansion is not always the objective. Preservation of ceiling across months and years often reflects deeper integration than rapid short-term change.

Intermittent fasting can be appropriate. When energy demand, sleep architecture, and recovery bandwidth align proportionately, it may reduce decision load, stabilize appetite rhythm, and support coherent oscillation. It can simplify feeding architecture without compressing margin.

It can also be misaligned. When stress density accumulates, sleep fragments, or workload escalates without corresponding restoration, identical structure may narrow bandwidth. The window itself is not the destabilizer; mismatch is. Recognizing this distinction requires decision clarity rather than intensity.

Structure differs from ideology. Ideology resists modification. Structure invites calibration. Calibration respects adaptive range and recovery margin. Escalation assumes that more intensity equals more progress. In biological systems, greater intensity without proportional restoration often reduces flexibility rather than enhancing it.

Signal coherence underpins long-horizon stability. Oscillation between fed and fasted states must remain recoverable. Recovery margin must exceed compression load. Adaptive bandwidth must be protected. These principles apply whether fasting is present or absent. Timing is one variable within a larger architecture.

Less intensity can produce more stability. A slightly wider margin may preserve oscillation amplitude over years, whereas aggressive compression may generate short-term movement followed by drift. Neutrality allows this trade-off to be evaluated without emotional distortion.

Identity attachment distorts interpretation. When fasting becomes proof of discipline or competence, adjustment feels like loss. Yet adaptive systems reward coherence, not symbolic consistency. Decision clarity emerges when structure is evaluated through context rather than defended through identity.

Long-horizon integration consistently outperforms short-term gains because biology integrates across cycles. Small misalignments repeated across months narrow margin more effectively than dramatic single events. Conversely, modest alignment sustained across seasons preserves capacity more reliably than aggressive compression maintained briefly.

Neutrality reduces volatility by removing moral charge from structure. Without moral overlay, feedback can be interpreted mechanistically rather than defensively. Appetite volatility, sleep drift, plateau, or recovery lag become informational signals rather than threats to identity.

A tool remains neutral because it does not demand loyalty. It operates within parameters and yields outcomes relative to context. Doctrine, by contrast, resists modification. When intermittent fasting shifts from adjustable architecture to defended identity, calibration becomes difficult. Signals that indicate mismatch are reframed as personal failure rather than environmental information. Escalation replaces interpretation.

Biological systems reward coherence over intensity. Oscillation between feeding and fasting must remain recoverable. The depth of fasting must be matched by the density of restoration. When oscillation amplitude exceeds available recovery bandwidth, contraction follows. When amplitude fits within bandwidth, stability persists. The difference is rarely visible in a single week. It emerges across seasons.

Long-horizon integration depends less on maximizing any single variable and more on sustaining proportional relationships. Feeding timing, workload, sleep, and stress must remain dynamically aligned. A structure that integrates smoothly during one life phase may require recalibration in another. Neutrality allows recalibration without ideological friction.

"No escalation" does not mean "no intensity." It means intensity must remain proportional to restoration capacity. Expansion is possible when surplus bandwidth exists. Preservation becomes primary when bandwidth narrows. In both cases, structure functions best when it remains responsive rather than rigid.

Intermittent fasting does not need defense. It needs context. It can coexist with stability for decades when aligned proportionately. It can narrow margin when layered onto misalignment. The variable is not the clock itself, but the coherence between timing and total load.

Intermittent fasting, then, is neither inherently corrective nor inherently destabilizing. It is an adjustable temporal framework. Its value depends on whether it supports recoverable oscillation, preserves recovery margin, and aligns proportionately with evolving demand.

Intermittent fasting is a contextual structural tool whose effectiveness depends on proportional alignment, adaptive bandwidth, and long-horizon coherence rather than on intensity, escalation, or identity attachment.

Readers interested in deeper exploration of fasting physiology may continue with *Fasting Fundamentals*, which examines extended fasting durations, metabolic transitions, and recovery considerations in greater detail.

About the Author

Nathan Reed writes about metabolic stability in systems exposed to load, variability, and time.

His work examines how biological capacity is shaped by energy availability, recovery architecture, sleep amplitude, muscle mass, environmental demand and workload. Rather than treating nutrition, fasting, sleep, and training as isolated tactics, he approaches them as interacting regulatory systems governed by margin, buffering, oscillatory coherence, and constraint dominance.

The Stability framework explores how physiological compression accumulates gradually and how proportional calibration preserves long-horizon resilience across decades. The objective is not peak optimization, but preservation of functional continuity under load.

Intermittent Fasting is part of a broader metabolic stability ecosystem developed under Perennial Publishing, each volume addressing a distinct vector of biological durability.

The work is designed for readers who prefer structural clarity over motivational rhetoric and long-horizon coherence over short-term intensity.

The Metabolic Stability Series

Metabolic Stability: A Systems Guide to Blood Sugar, Fasting, and Long-Term Metabolic Health

(Cornerstone Volume)

Fasting Fundamentals

(Foundational Volume)

Intermittent Fasting

Future Titles Include:

Prolonged Fasting

Insulin Stability

Electrolytes

Sleep and Recovery (Vitality Series)

Strength and Aging (Vitality Series)

Part of a Broader Stability Framework

The Metabolic Stability Series is part of a larger stability ecosystem published by Perennial Publishing.

Related domains include:

Money Stability — structural durability in financial systems

Career Stability — positioning, load tolerance, and transition resilience

Mental Stability — cognitive steadiness under pressure and uncertainty

Emotional Stability — regulatory steadiness in environments that do not slow down

Foundations (Foundational Living Systems) — low-fragility life architecture

Each domain approaches stability as a structural problem: capacity versus load, buffering versus shock, governance versus drift. Together, they form a unified framework for long-horizon durability across the major systems that shape human trajectory.

For bulk or institutional orders, contact Perennial Publishing.